Bev Aisbett is the author and illustrator of 15 highly regarded self-help texts for sufferers of anxiety and depression, most notably *Living with IT* and *Taming the Black Dog*. These books are distributed to health professionals nationwide and have been translated into four languages.

A trained counsellor, Bev is also the facilitator of the *Art of Anxiety* recovery program in Melbourne. For those unable to attend her workshop in person, she offers a home-study version, *The Art of Anxiety DVD Workshop*, as well as other online resources and services. She conducts lectures to assist sufferers of depression and anxiety within metropolitan and regional Victoria.

Bev is also a recognised artist, and her soulful paintings have been regularly exhibited in Victoria and Tasmania.

Workshop and lecture information,
and other anxiety resources:
www.bevaisbettartofanxiety.com

BY BEV AISBETT

Living IT Up

Letting IT Go

Get Real

Taming the Black Dog

The Little Book of IT

Fixing IT

Recovery: A Journey to Healing

The Book of IT

Get Over IT

I Love Me

All of IT: A Memoir

Living with IT

30 Days 30 Ways to Overcome Anxiety

30 Days 30 Ways to Overcome Depression

Worry-Proofing Your Anxious Child

WORRY-PROOFING YOUR ANXIOUS CHILD

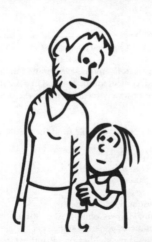

BEV AISBETT

HarperCollins*Publishers*

HarperCollins_Publishers_
Australia • Brazil • Canada • France • Germany • Holland • Hungary
India • Italy • Japan • Mexico • New Zealand • Poland • Spain • Sweden
Switzerland • United Kingdom • United States of America

First published in Australia in 2020
by HarperCollins_Publishers_ Australia Pty Limited
ABN 36 009 913 517
harpercollins.com.au

A catalogue record for this book is available from the National Library of Australia.

ISBN 978 1 4607 5719 2 (paperback)
ISBN 978 1 4607 1095 1 (ebook)
ISBN 978 1 4607 9435 7 (audiobook)

Cover and internal illustrations by Bev Aisbett
Cover design by Hazel Lam, HarperCollins Design Studio
Typeset in Brandon Grotesque by Kelli Lonergan
Printed and bound in Australia by McPherson's Printing Group
The papers used by HarperCollins in the manufacture of this book are a natural,
recyclable product made from wood grown in sustainable plantation forests. The fibre
source and manufacturing processes meet recognised international environmental
standards, and carry certification.

DEDICATION

To my parents –
who did their best for
their anxious child

CONTENTS

INTRODUCTION

First up, this is not a book on PARENTING.

My expertise is not in that field. So I'm going to assume that you're doing the best job at being a parent as any normal, flawed human being can.

In other words, you'll get it right sometimes and sometimes you won't, and that's okay. You're doing the best that you know how, but a little extra LEARNING always comes in handy, yes?

Parenting is a tough and tricky job, and sometimes there are extra CHALLENGES that make it seem even harder, such as having a child who is anxious.

What I am an expert on is this thing called ANXIETY, and this book is designed to help you UNDERSTAND it so that you can help your child deal with their own anxiety.

My approach is not necessarily a conventional one. The focus is not on this being a big, hairy problem, so much as NOT MAKING IT into a big, hairy problem!

For a start, I find any message unhelpful that says that someone is STUCK with anxiety.

To my mind and in my own personal experience of anxiety, it is more of a reactive approach to life's ups and downs than a 'condition'.

So, you'll find that I'm not big on protecting your children from anxiety as much as teaching them how not to FEAR it. It (or **IT**, as anxiety is known in my other books) is not a MONSTER but a part of the self that needs some reining in, soothing and direction.

There is no greater motivator than anxiety to force POSITIVE and NECESSARY changes to one's approach to life.

If this opportunity is seized – if the HEALTHY changes become the FOCUS instead of the anxiety – the REWARDS can last a lifetime.

With these new LIFE SKILLS in place, anxiety ceases to be all-consuming and, in time and with PRACTICE, can become a non-issue and even a helpful asset.

My aim is to show you and your little worrier how to make that happen.

GETTING HELP FOR YOUR CHILD

While the approaches in this book are designed to help guide you in assisting your child, if the child's anxiety remains OVERWHELMING and ONGOING, it may be necessary to seek PROFESSIONAL HELP.

This does not necessarily mean that your child's anxiety is more SERIOUS than normal, but they may simply need to explore issues on a more PERSONAL level.

There are situations where a child's anxiety is affecting them to a SIGNIFICANT level or their anxiety has arisen out of genuine TRAUMA, and these will most certainly require professional attention.

A good place to begin is to speak with your child's teachers or the school counsellor about how your child is COPING, and ask about the type of SUPPORT they would recommend. Also, you can have a conversation with your GP about getting a referral to see a therapist and possibly set up a mental health care plan.

Choosing the right THERAPIST for your child is a significant choice because this person will act as an ALLY, CONFIDANT and FRIEND to your child.

The child needs to feel CONFIDENT in their therapist and that they can TRUST them enough to share their deepest fears and feelings. It is therefore important that you INCLUDE your child in choosing the appropriate therapist for them.

Ideally, give the RELATIONSHIP a chance to grow, rather than making a decision after just one session. Two or three sessions may be enough to determine COMPATABILITY and whether there is PROGRESS, and ask your child to give you feedback along the way so you can UNDERSTAND how they're feeling.

CHAPTER 1

Is this NORMAL?

I think my child
has **ANXIETY**!
I'm really **WORRIED**
for her!

Okay, BOTH of you
worrying isn't going
to HELP, is it?

ANXIETY itself
is NORMAL!

It's an
EVOLUTIONARY
HANGOVER
that is part of
our SURVIVAL
INSTINCT.

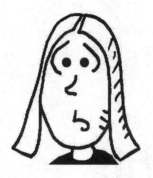

This goes back to ancient times when we had to be
ALERT to any potential DANGER, such as:

PREDATORS

ENEMIES

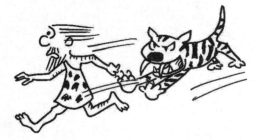

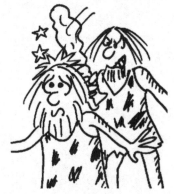

SHORTAGE OF SURVIVAL NEEDS

PHYSICAL DANGERS

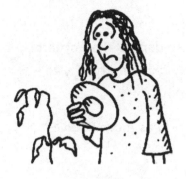

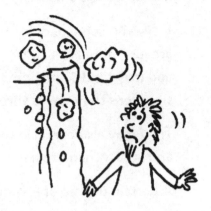

And probably most significantly, as this is STILL a primary factor in anxiety:

REJECTION BY THE 'TRIBE'

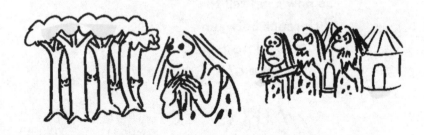

If the tribe evicted you, you were in greater DANGER without the protection that the tribe afforded against the ELEMENTS, STARVATION or PREDATORS.

We'll explore this last point in some detail later, but sensitivity to potential DANGER is common to most human beings and is an essential tool for our SURVIVAL.

However, some people, including some CHILDREN, are just more HYPERVIGILANT to danger than others and may tend to react more quickly or strongly to situations they see as threatening.

They may also perceive the world as more DANGEROUS and SCARY than others.

A certain degree of FEAR is normal in children as they encounter new situations (which is also true for ADULTS, is it not?), but this usually disappears once they become familiar and comfortable with the situation.

So how can I tell the difference between ANXIETY and NORMAL WORRYING?

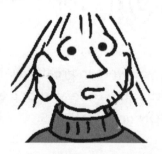

There are several telltale signs that may indicate ANXIETY.

Is your child excessively:

SEEKING REASSURANCE?

I'M OKAY, YOU'RE OKAY, IT'S ALL OKAY ... I'M OKAY, YOU'RE OKAY, IT'S ALL OKAY ...

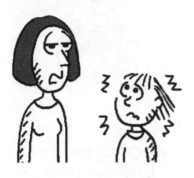

AVOIDING INTERACTIONS/ ACTIVITIES?

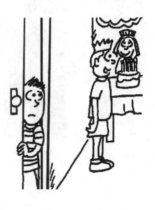

INVENTING ILLNESSES?

Again?

My tummy HURTS!

TRYING TO GET YOU TO DO THINGS FOR THEM?

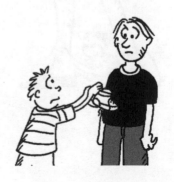

AVOIDING TAKING RISKS OR TRYING NEW THINGS?

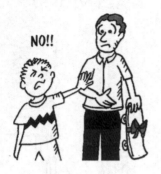

WORRYING/ FRETTING?

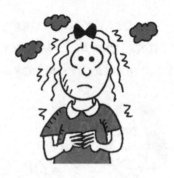

BEING CLINGY?

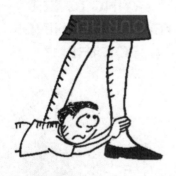

EMOTIONAL OVER MINOR UPSETS?

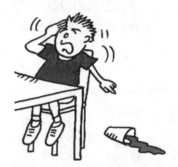

RELUCTANT TO GO TO SCHOOL?

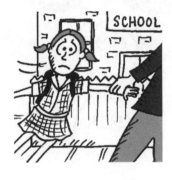

AFRAID TO SLEEP ALONE?

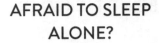
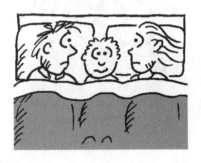

SHY OR NERVOUS AROUND OTHERS?

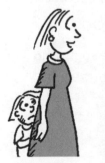
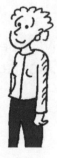

SCARED OF NUMEROUS THINGS?

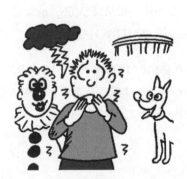

COMPLAINING OF BEING PICKED ON?

NEGATIVE IN OUTLOOK?

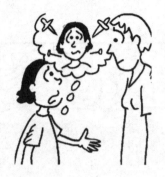
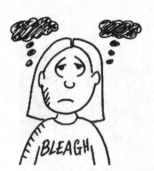

If your child is excessively doing some of these things, then it is likely that ANXIETY may be a problem for them.

Most commonly, children experiencing anxiety will DOUBT THEMSELVES, lack CONFIDENCE and become easily OVERWHELMED.

In general, they are HIGHLY SENSITIVE little souls who tend to OVERREACT, DRAMATISE, EXAGGERATE and think in EXTREMES.

My child tends to WORRY a lot! Does that mean she'll develop ANXIETY?

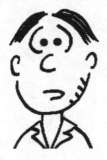

Most people worry at some time or other, but not everyone who worries develops ANXIETY.

However, in those more PREDISPOSED to anxiety, excessive and even compulsive worrying is the FUEL that FEEDS anxiety.

But here's the thing, that's just like ANXIOUS ADULTS.

Which raises the question: do we LEARN to be anxious or is it INNATE? (More on that in CHAPTER 4: NATURE OR NURTURE?)

CHAPTER 2

ANXIETY 101

**So what IS anxiety?
I have to admit that
I don't really GET it!**

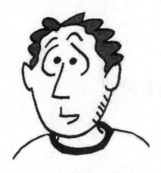

Anxiety is a state of
HYPERVIGILANCE, when
the natural inner 'ALARM'
that keeps us alert
to danger (and thereby
assists our survival)
STAYS on the alert
for danger or perceives
danger, even WHEN
THERE IS NONE.

It's a SURVIVAL INSTINCT that has gone into OVERDRIVE.

This can also mean that there is an OVERREACTION
to even MINOR threats, such as RUNNING LATE or
being CRITICISED.

**But why the big drama?
My child's LIFE
isn't in danger!**

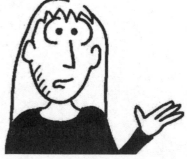

But the child's EGO feels threatened. You know that little INNER VOICE that we all have, that gives an ongoing 'report' about EVERYTHING we do? That's the EGO talking.

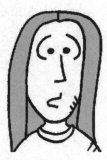

Why do we have an INNER VOICE at all?

Basically, the mind, as EGO, needs to VALIDATE itself ...

I'm HERE!
I MATTER!

... and by REPORTING ourselves to ourselves, the EGO affirms that yep, I still exist.

Here I AM,
DOING THIS
now!

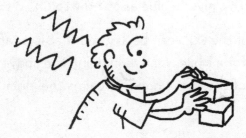

This inner voice gives a clue to the origins of ANXIETY. Anxiety arises when the EGO is under threat. We see evidence of this when we place so much importance on others' opinions of us and on a fear of 'failing'.

I'm INVISIBLE!

The big fear for the EGO is ANNIHILATION, i.e., not existing, and so it goes into SURVIVAL MODE when faced with potential 'extinction'.

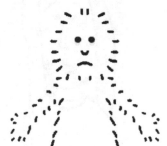

And, of course, children (especially very young children) are by nature EGOCENTRIC and remain so until the full DEVELOPMENT of the brain, which is not complete until the AGE OF 25!

However, the EGO (presenting as that inner voice) disappears now and then when we are totally ABSORBED in something or in DEEP MEDITATION. This gives a clue as to how to CALM the inner voice.

If the EGO can be assured that it is safe to 'disappear' for a while, such as in doing the above, then doing more of the above not only calms the inner chatter but also takes us out of ourselves and away from the need to have our EXISTENCE and WORTH affirmed every minute.

Even so, anxiety can feel very OVERWHELMING, especially in the initial stages. It's not easy to FUNCTION, and your child may do ANYTHING to avoid experiencing those feelings.

There is a feeling of UNREALITY with anxiety.

FAMILIAR things can seem suddenly SINISTER or THREATENING.

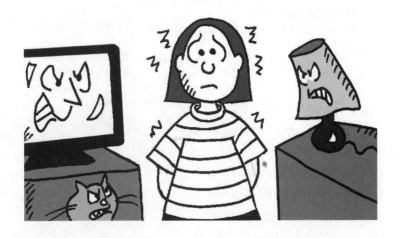

There is a feeling of DREAD. Just being CONSCIOUS can seem SCARY. There is a feeling that something BAD is going to happen, despite evidence to the CONTRARY.

The PHYSICAL SYMPTOMS of anxiety can include:

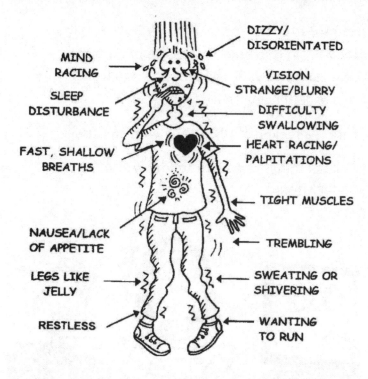

MIND RACING

SLEEP DISTURBANCE

FAST, SHALLOW BREATHS

NAUSEA/LACK OF APPETITE

LEGS LIKE JELLY

RESTLESS

DIZZY/ DISORIENTATED

VISION STRANGE/BLURRY

DIFFICULTY SWALLOWING

HEART RACING/ PALPITATIONS

TIGHT MUSCLES

TREMBLING

SWEATING OR SHIVERING

WANTING TO RUN

However, as DRAMATIC and INTENSE as these symptoms may seem when seen as a package, they are still just NORMAL RESPONSES to one thing – FEAR.

Where does this fear come from? Our home is SAFE! We are a LOVING FAMILY!

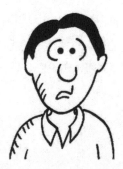

The FEAR your child is experiencing is most likely only marginally based on ACTUAL threats that have become EXAGGERATED in the child's mind.

Their THOUGHTS are running a little WILD, and they need to learn how to TRAIN them. Getting your THINKING right is the key to managing and overcoming anxiety.

When we perceive threats, our NORMAL INSTINCTS tell us to do one of two things – FIGHT or FLEE.

Again, this is a PRIMAL, SURVIVAL-BASED response. It's in our HARDWIRING.

It goes back to our ancient roots when, if confronted with danger, such as wild predators, we could either stay and FIGHT or RUN AWAY.

What is really happening when we have this response is the BODY and MIND PREPARING us to deal with the DANGER.

This PHYSIOLOGICAL REACTION is designed to HELP US!

Several things happen when our system goes through this process. We will look at this in detail later, but the diagram of SYMPTOMS on page 20 gives you the general picture.

When someone experiences these PHYSICAL SENSATIONS, they are interpreted as meaning that there is something to be AFRAID OF. However, the symptoms themselves are not 'proof' of an actual THREAT; rather, they indicate an IDEA of a threat.

Naturally, if we FEEL scared, we look for REASONS why we feel scared and we create a 'story' to EXPLAIN the sensations, such as:

When people don't LIKE you, it's SCARY.

Mum being SICK is SCARY.

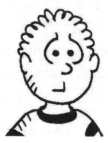
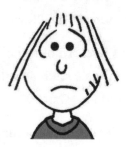

In doing so, we assign power to OBJECTS, EVENTS or PEOPLE to 'MAKE' us anxious, when, in fact, this is just a STORY that we have attached to explain feelings of discomfort.

A common definition of this phenomenon is 'A CATASTROPHIC MISINTERPRETATION OF PHYSICAL SENSATIONS'.

It is important to keep in mind that children –
especially very YOUNG children – have yet to develop
the ability to REASON, so even minor upsets, by
adult standards, may be interpreted as much more
significant to the child.

If someone experiencing anxiety can learn to 'RIDE
OUT' the physical sensations without making too
much of them, the feelings will pass more quickly.

Remember that the symptoms themselves are not
'proof' of an actual THREAT; they indicate an IDEA of
a threat and that one's THINKING is out of balance.

Aside from the PHYSICAL SYMPTOMS, there are also
changes that happen in the BRAIN in response to FEAR.

THIS IS THE AMYGDALA

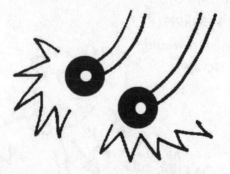

This is the part of the brain that processes STRONG
EMOTIONS.

Normally, once the 'danger' has passed, the system resets; but if there is a constant FOCUS on anxious thoughts or even fear of the anxiety itself, 'danger' is still being registered and the amygdala remains STIMULATED.

So, if we analyse this, nothing BAD is actually happening! The real fear is an ANTICIPATION of danger or an EXAGGERATION of apparent danger. The only thing that needs to change is the default position of FEARFUL THOUGHTS, and the rest will follow!

The difference between GARDEN-VARIETY anxiety and CHRONIC anxiety is simply ONGOING FOCUS and ATTENTION given to the ANXIETY! Being ANXIOUS, or FEELING BAD in general, can become a HABIT.

I HATE this!
It's HORRIBLE!
I wish it would
GO AWAY!

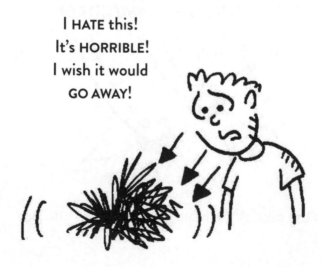

Imagine that anxiety is a plant that is fed by anxious or fearful THOUGHTS, which include anxious thoughts about the anxiety itself. The more you feed anxiety with FEAR (i.e., the more you FOCUS on it), the BIGGER it grows!

Along with the fear is an inner monologue that is CRITICAL, PESSIMISTIC and PUNISHING.

You're an IDIOT! You always MESS THINGS UP! You'll NEVER get it right! Everybody's LOOKING at you!

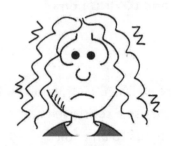

This inner voice is ever-watchful for ways that the person might mess up and therefore be JUDGED as LACKING. Its criticism is really aimed at PROTECTING the self from making a MISTAKE that may place them in peril.

Both the fear of possible danger and the fear of being judged go back to our evolutionary roots, as we will explore more in CHAPTER 4: NATURE OR NURTURE?

The FEAR OF DANGER helps to protect us from natural threats. The NEED TO BELONG provides us with the safety of the tribe.

These are very PRIMAL and PRIMITIVE instincts, which can be triggered by situations and events that FEEL traumatic.

But my child hasn't been exposed to TRAUMA! We have a SAFE and LOVING home!

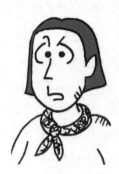

We're all DIFFERENT, and the things that may traumatise a sensitive child may appear to be fairly innocuous to an adult.*

This is because as adults, we learn to RATIONALISE or REASON.

---

*Of course, there are circumstances of anxiety arising from genuine trauma. In this case, PROFESSIONAL HELP is necessary. Please see 'GETTING HELP FOR YOUR CHILD' on pages 3–4.

A child does not have those points of reference, so 'trauma' may be as apparently 'minor' as:

A BOISTEROUS DOG

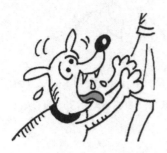

BEING TEASED

BEING ALONE

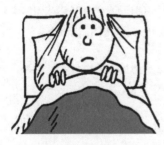

LIFE CHANGES

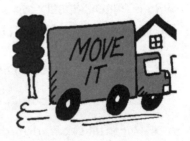

GOOD GRIEF!
Does that mean we have to wrap her in **COTTON WOOL?**

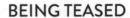

ABSOLUTELY NOT!

This will only CONFIRM the idea that there is something to be AFRAID of.

27

But my child gets so DISTRESSED! It's hard to just STAND by!

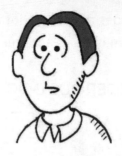

Anxiety is no FUN, that's for sure. It can feel very, very SCARY, but again, in general, NOTHING BAD IS ACTUALLY HAPPENING!

However, there are certain LIFE CHANGES and CHALLENGES that can be anxiety-provoking in a child who is PREDISPOSED towards anxious responses (just as these things can trigger anxiety in ADULTS, too):

- Moving house or to a new country
- Change of school
- Parental separation/divorce
- Death or illness in the family
- Illness or disability in the child
- Changes in friendships
- Bullying
- Abuse and neglect
- Natural disasters

Some of these things are UNAVOIDABLE in life.

What can I DO?

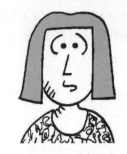

That is the POINT. Life brings with it INEVITABLE CHALLENGES. Your priority is not so much to PROTECT your child from the UPS and DOWNS that life throws at us, but to teach them that they are UP TO THE CHALLENGE.

Life is TOUGH. You need to EQUIP your child to HANDLE it with poise and confidence, rather than FEARING the challenges that life brings.

This doesn't mean BEING tough (as in RUTHLESS or UNCARING); it means being RESILIENT and FLEXIBLE.

Never-ending HAPPINESS and COMFORT are not NATURAL states. There are cycles of WELLBEING and cycles of CHALLENGES.

Kids are not FRAIL, DELICATE flowers – unless they are TAUGHT to be. Get a kid ANGRY, and you'll see what a MYTH that is!

And even very young children have their own WISDOM, if you encourage them to look for it and are open to hearing it.

They are able to solve PROBLEMS if you give them the opportunity to come up with their own SOLUTIONS.

And the things that BUG you are the same things that bug your kids.

Do you like:

- HAVING to do something?
- Being told what to DO?
- Being endlessly SCRUTINISED?
- Being told how you FEEL?

Anxious people – children and adults alike – have the following traits in COMMON:

Anxious people tend to EXTREMES –they don't have small PROBLEMS, they have CATASTROPHES.

Oh NO!
It's a
DISASTER!

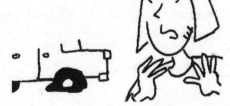

They don't have LOSSES, they have TRAGEDIES.

I lost my JOB!

I thought you HATED it!

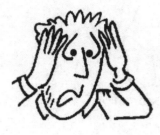 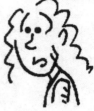

They have savage INNER CRITICS.

You're such an IDIOT!
Who could LOVE you?

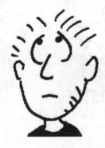

They are fearful of MAKING MISTAKES.

Don't BLOW it!

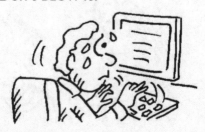

They worry about how they are PERCEIVED.

A coffee stain!
What will they
THINK?

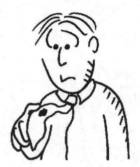

They look OUTSIDE themselves for WISDOM and GUIDANCE.

Tell me what
to DO!

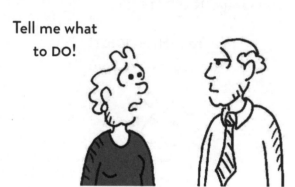

They are DEPENDENT.

Don't LEAVE me!

I'm just checking
THE MAIL!

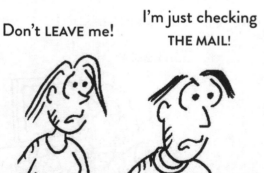

They don't TRUST themselves.

I just KNOW
I'll MESS IT UP!

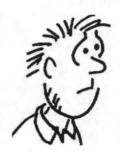

They have an UNHELPFUL THINKING STYLE.

WRONG! BAD!
WORRY!
WHAT IF?
TOO HARD!

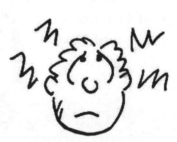

Their worries are mostly FUTURE-BASED.

What if the bridge
FALLS DOWN?

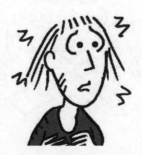

They tend to be PEOPLE-PLEASERS.

Please LIKE ME!

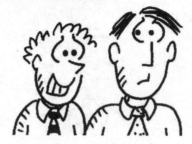

They lean towards PERFECTIONISM.

Oh NO! A CREASE!
I'll have to
CHANGE clothes!

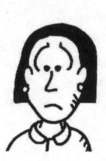

They are often HIGH ACHIEVERS.

PUSH, PUSH, PUSH!

CHAPTER 3

What's going on UPSTAIRS

**So how does
one get INTO
this anxious
state?**

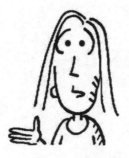

By THINKING in an
ANXIOUS way!

An event might occur that a child INTERPRETS as being
SCARY. This creates a FEAR response, which sets off a
CHEMICAL REACTION in the BRAIN.

In response, the body prepares itself for the best
course of action for SURVIVAL, which, as we saw earlier,
may mean FIGHT or FLIGHT.

The FIGHT-OR-FLIGHT response refers to a physiological
reaction that occurs in the presence of something that
is interpreted as being a THREAT, either MENTALLY or
PHYSICALLY.

Hormones are released that prepare the body either to STAY and DEAL WITH the threat or to RUN AWAY to safety.

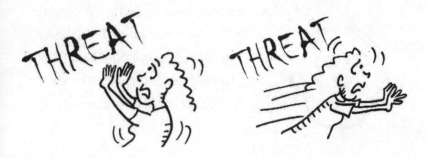

The PHYSIOLOGICAL changes that occur include:

• RAPID HEARTBEAT AND BREATHING

Heartbeat and respiration rates increase to ensure that the body has the ENERGY and OXYGEN it needs to either run or fight in response to the danger.

• PALE OR FLUSHED SKIN

As blood flow increases to the MUSCLES, BRAIN, LEGS and ARMS, the face may alternate between appearing PALE, as blood moves away to the limbs, or FLUSHED, as blood rushes back to the head and brain.

• DILATED PUPILS

Dilation of the pupils allows more light into the eyes and results in BETTER VISION of the surroundings. This allows in more VISUAL INFORMATION to help us determine the best action for self-preservation.

• TREMBLING

MUSCLES become tense so as to be primed for action. This tension can result in TREMBLING or SHAKING.

The above physiological changes are all perfectly NATURAL responses to DANGER. They are the body/brain's way of aiding SURVIVAL.

Once the danger has passed, everything can reset – or should – UNLESS there remains a thought that DANGER is still present ...

... which is where the MIND comes in.

The VITAL CLUE to the true nature of anxiety and why anxiety can become an ONGOING problem is:

ANXIOUS THINKING

Let's take a look at what's going on UPSTAIRS as a result of having ANXIOUS THOUGHTS.

Something happens (or perhaps SEVERAL things over a period of time) that generates a FEAR RESPONSE. This is processed in an area of the brain that deals with strong emotions, the AMYGDALA. The amygdala signals the brain to set in motion the PHYSIOLOGICAL responses that we just examined.

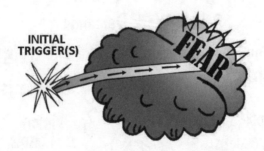

Normally, once the 'DANGER' has passed, everything can RESET and you can CALM DOWN ...

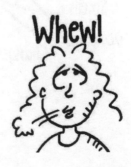

WATCH OUT!

... but if you think there's still something to FEAR, you'll stay on ALERT ...

... and if you REMAIN on alert, it will take FEWER stimuli to set off this REACTION.

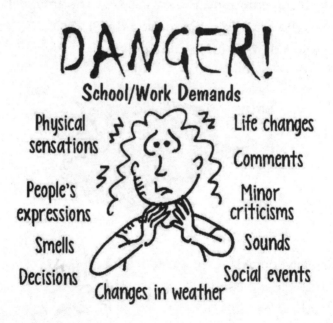

DANGER!

School/Work Demands

Physical sensations

Life changes

Comments

People's expressions

Minor criticisms

Smells

Sounds

Decisions

Social events

Changes in weather

As more and more FEAR RESPONSES occur, a BRIDGE in the BRAIN starts to form that goes DIRECTLY to RED ALERT, even after a minor TRIGGER.

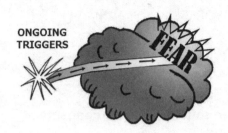

When someone learns to respond CALMLY to triggers, a NEW BRIDGE takes them to a new, better-feeling part of the BRAIN.

And the MORE OFTEN one takes oneself there (with CALMING, SUPPORTIVE or REASSURING thoughts), the STRONGER this new bridge will become, and the old bridge will begin to FALL AWAY.

This actually
changes the way
the BRAIN WORKS!

AMAZING, yes?

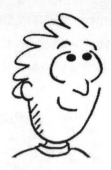

Here we see some ESSENTIAL concepts:

- Anxiety has less to do with EXTERNAL EVENTS
  and more to do with the way these events are
  INTERPRETED and PROCESSED.

- THOUGHTS can either ADD to anxiety or EASE it.

- While we may not have control over external
  events, we have control of the way we RESPOND
  to them.

- Things can either feel BAD or GOOD, depending
  on how we REPORT them to ourselves.

- Someone can change the way something FEELS
  by how they THINK about it – therefore, the
  experience of REALITY is changed.

- Someone can feel GOOD or BAD about something BEFORE it actually happens, which will affect their experience of it when it does happen.

- Something is only as SCARY / BAD / AWFUL as someone THINKS it is!

Getting THINKING right is THE way to change, not only anxiety but pretty much EVERYTHING!

Here are a few ways to address unhelpful thinking:

1. AVOID ABSOLUTES

ABSOLUTES override any sense of FREE CHOICE. They create PRESSURE, and there is no MIDDLE GROUND.

Here are the main culprits:

'SHOULD!'
'MUST!'
'HAVE TO!'
'GOT TO!'

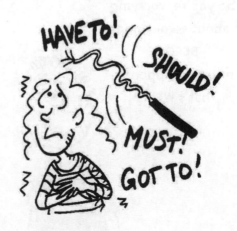

Introduce the idea of CHOICE and the pressure eases.

I CHOOSE to go.

Well, I PREFER to stay!

 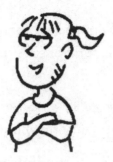

2. STAY IN THE PRESENT

Anxiety is mainly based on POTENTIAL and, therefore, FUTURE-BASED worries. Staying focused in the PRESENT means less WORRYING.

So you're worrying about something **BEFORE** it even happens? That's WEIRD!

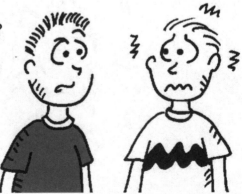

3. WHAT IF?

What if?
What if?
What if?

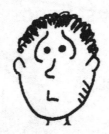

THE mantra for anxiety is 'What if?'

- *What if I fail?*

- *What if I make a fool of myself?*

- *What if they don't like me?*

- *What if it all goes wrong?*

There is a simple REMEDY to the question 'What if?' – and that is to ANSWER it.

Okay, let's say you
DID fail the test,
what ELSE could
you do if that happens?

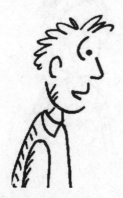

Hmm, I guess
I could take the
test AGAIN!

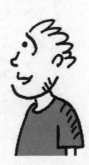

4. THINGS ARE JUST THINGS

It's a
HORRIBLE
day!

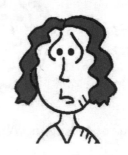

No, it isn't. It's just a DAY that you THINK is
horrible. Change your OPINION and the day
will feel DIFFERENT!

5. THOUGHTS ARE NOT FACTS

I'm a **BAD PERSON!**
Everything is going
to go **WRONG!**
Everyone will think
I'm **STUPID!**

Gee, where do you
get your **INFO?**

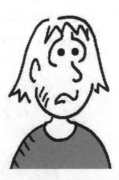

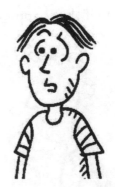

6. EXPLORE OTHER OPTIONS

What's a BETTER WAY
to THINK about this?

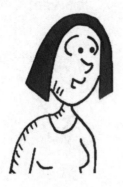 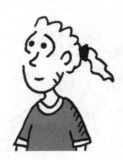

7. GET SUPER CHOOSY!

NO
NEGATIVITY,
PUT-DOWNS,
MEAN STUFF
OR SCARY IDEAS
ALLOWED

Oh, I'm VERY
PICKY about the
THOUGHTS
I entertain!

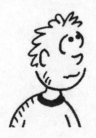 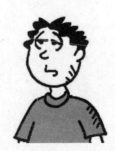

8. STICK TO THE FACTS

It's a
DISASTER!

No – it's a
PROBLEM to be
SOLVED!

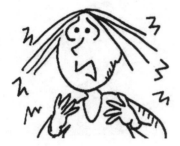 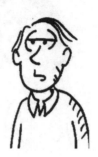

9. BE NICE

HOW you think or talk about something has a HUGE impact on how it FEELS to you.

Consciously thinking and speaking CALMLY and KINDLY about situations, others and yourself can have an equally CALMING effect on your MOOD.

CHAPTER 4

NATURE or NURTURE?

Are anxious people BORN that way or do they LEARN to be anxious?

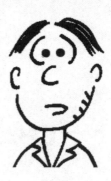

Actually, it's a bit of BOTH. Just as some people are born with certain PHYSICAL CHALLENGES, others may be born with PSYCHOLOGICAL or EMOTIONAL CHALLENGES. In either case, this does not CONDEMN anyone to defined limitations but may require greater MANAGEMENT, and this is especially true of ANXIETY.

Studies on the NATURE/NURTURE question have revealed some common factors with regard to a propensity to ANXIETY.

Let's start with NATURE.

People with anxiety are often:

- **GOOD WITH WORDS**

Mother, I'm feeling
a little PERTURBED today!

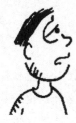
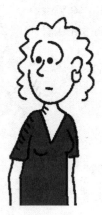

This may mean a more HEIGHTENED or 'elaborate'
experience and recall of events – especially
UNPLEASANT events.

In other words, anxious people may tend to be
'STUCK IN THEIR HEADS' and experience things more
INTENSELY, ruminating on the PAST and speculating
on the FUTURE in great detail.

• HAVE A HIGHER I.Q.

You only worry because you're so SMART!

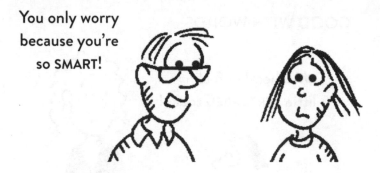

Yes, there is some evidence that the SMARTER you are the more prone you may be to experiencing ANXIETY.

Again, this may be down to EVOLUTION – the quicker you THINK, the quicker you are to REACT for your own survival. However, this also means being constantly on the lookout for potential DANGER, even where none currently exists.

• FEMALE

The gender divide here is not entirely STRAIGHTFORWARD, with teenage girls and women tending to be more anxious.

It's a **MAN'S WORLD** out there.

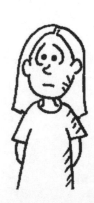

Males may actually be MORE anxious up to age 11, but by age 15 the trend is REVERSED.

Why girls become more anxious as they age may be explained by HORMONES, but there is a strong argument that different SOCIALISATION between girls and boys may be a key factor.

Aw, she's shy.
Isn't that SWEET?

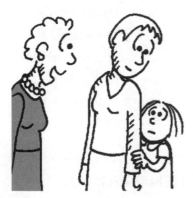

Don't be such
a WUSS!

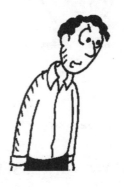

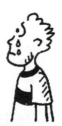

Anxious people may also have:

• MORE ACTIVE PROCESSING CENTRES IN THE BRAIN

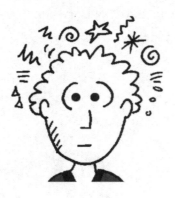

... in particular, the AMYGDALA, the region of the brain that processes strong emotion, such as FEAR. (We've looked at the role of the amygdala previously, in CHAPTER 2: ANXIETY 101.)

It may also be that:

• MUM WAS STRESSED WHEN PREGNANT

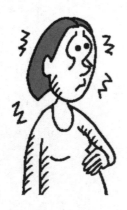

The natural barrier between the placenta and the foetus that protects the baby from STRESS HORMONES in the mother's blood can become ineffective if the mother is highly stressed during pregnancy.

And some of us are just:

- **BORN SENSITIVE**

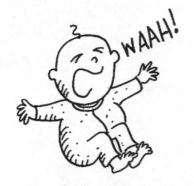

We're all DIFFERENT and that includes our HARDWIRING! Babies easily upset by strange NOISES, TOYS or SMELLS tend to remain SENSITIVE into adulthood.

There is also some evidence that a predisposition to anxiety may be part of a GENETIC INHERITANCE, which means that certain FAMILY GROUPS may be more predisposed to anxiety than others.

However, although these individuals may be more INCLINED to being fretful, this doesn't mean they are DOOMED to be! This simply means that they need to be more AWARE of their sensitivity and reduce their exposure to STRESSORS – especially STRESSFUL THINKING!

With the RIGHT SKILLS, anyone can learn to be more relaxed. While there may not be a lot you can do about PREDISPOSING FACTORS, there is a lot you CAN do about how this turns out.

Now let's look at the NURTURE ASPECT.

Children are little SPONGES, soaking up the experience of life in huge amounts (especially in their early years) and learning mostly from their CARETAKERS.

CHILDHOOD is a time when we LEARN:

- **WHAT TO EXPECT FROM LIFE**

  Life's a STRUGGLE!   Life's GOOD!

  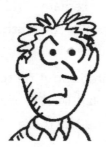   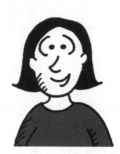

- **WHAT LOVE FEELS LIKE**

  I'll love you   I love you
  if you BEHAVE!   UNCONDITIONALLY!

  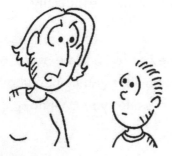   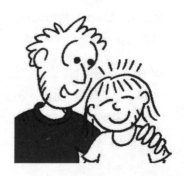

• HOW POWERFUL PEOPLE INTERACT

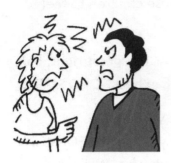 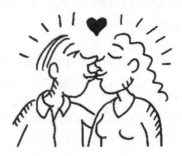

Children learn mostly by OBSERVATION. WORDS don't teach. ACTIONS, ATTITUDES and INTENTIONS do.

A child will pick up on your VIBE faster than your WORDS.

Showing children how to DEAL with challenges offers them more practical life skills than PROTECTING them from challenges.

Okay kids – watch how I HANDLE this!

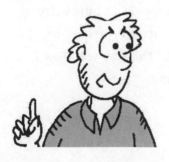 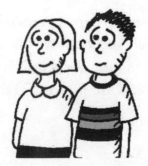

PARENTING STYLES

Certain parenting styles can cause children to feel INSECURE.

Parenting can be a BALANCING ACT to get it right, but UNDERSTANDING how it works can be a GOOD START.

While it's vitally important that you remain AUTHENTIC, it is also helpful for you to be INFORMED and to MODIFY behaviours that may be UNHELPFUL.

EXAMINING your approach can also give you insights into any sticking points you may have because of the way YOU were parented, and allow you to adopt a healthier approach, not only for the sake of your children, but also for YOURSELF.

Often, we have inherited ATTITUDES and BELIEFS that are passed down, unexamined, through several generations, so in fact you may be parenting in the same way as your GREAT-GRANDPARENTS did, without realising it!

The way we are parented in CHILDHOOD sends strong signals about our WORTH and ability to HANDLE life, and, in turn, these beliefs dictate the way we REACT or RESPOND in stressful situations.

Let's take a look at some UNHELPFUL PARENTING STYLES and the EMOTIONAL OUTCOMES they can produce:

- ## DISTANT

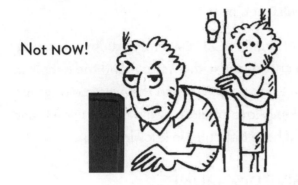

A parent being too BUSY, EMOTIONALLY UNAVAILABLE or UNDEMONSTRATIVE can send a message that the child is not of VALUE. The child may in turn create DRAMAS to gain the attention of the parent.

- ## ABUSIVE

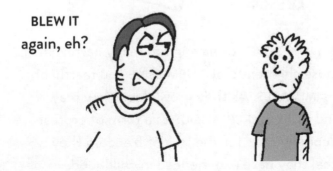

ABUSE can come in many forms – there is obvious abuse, involving VIOLENT and AGGRESSIVE behaviour, but EMOTIONAL ABUSE can include BELITTLING STATEMENTS, SARCASM or 'LOVE' given one minute, then WITHHELD the next.

Abuse, of ANY kind, is EXTREMELY destructive. It sends a message to children that the world – and the people in it – is UNSAFE and UNCARING. In the example of giving and withholding 'love', children will feel CONFUSED and UNSURE, and have difficulty in knowing who to TRUST.

• EXCESSIVE DISCIPLINE

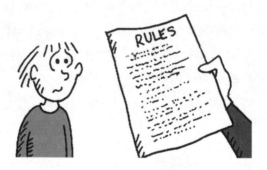

Being overly STRICT or having too many narrow RULES can cause children to be SUBMISSIVE and fearful of making MISTAKES. As they grow older, they may respond by being REBELLIOUS as a form of protest or to 'compensate' for the lack of freedom they may feel they have experienced in childhood.

• ANYTHING GOES

WHATEVER ...

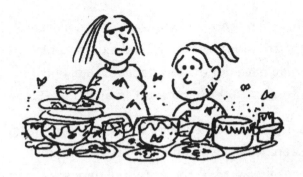

In contrast, an overly LAID-BACK, 'DO WHAT YOU LIKE' attitude can cause children to experience a lack of STRUCTURE and SECURITY. They may have trouble fitting in with SOCIETY'S CONVENTIONS and accepting RESPONSIBILITY. They will tend to blame OTHERS and OUTSIDE FACTORS for where they find themselves.

• SMOTHERING

On the other end of the spectrum, being OVERLY PROTECTIVE can teach children to DOUBT THEMSELVES and be overly reliant on others' APPROVAL, ADVICE and SUPPORT.

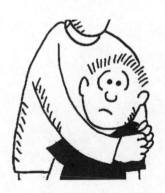

We have come a long way from the days of children being little more than INVISIBLE accoutrements or even 'servants'.

But we have also come a long way from children having the freedom to explore and experiment as they may have done a few decades ago, and to learn from MISTAKES and even small INJURIES.

As a result of access to a flood of information never before seen, we have an emerging parenting style that is acutely aware of the potential dangers of the world – anything from CLIMATE CHANGE and STRANGER DANGER to even UNHYGENIC KITCHEN SURFACES, which constitute the MYRIAD threats that are broadcast to us daily through the media and advertising.

It is important to note that while the world may APPEAR to be a more dangerous place, it may be the case that this is not necessarily so and that we are simply more AWARE of the dangers than ever before.

MODERN DANGERS	THE GOOD OLD DAYS

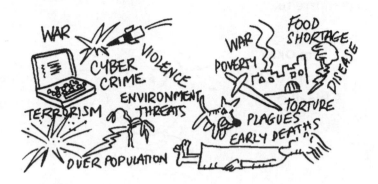

However, given the stream of threatening possibilities that we are subjected to, it is little wonder that parents can become overly CAUTIOUS – but this comes at a PRICE for your children.

While keeping your children SAFE may be your priority, there is a danger in being OVERLY protective.

Imagine arriving on Earth to begin your new and exciting adventure.

You're fresh as a DAISY and raring to go! You're not AFRAID – why would you be?

Bring it ON!

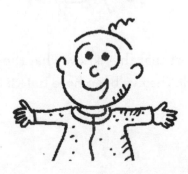

You have no JUDGMENT of anything or anyone (including YOURSELF), because you have nothing to compare to.

I'm OKAY.
You're OKAY.
It's all OKAY!

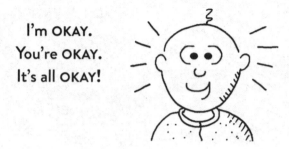

There are some POWERFUL GIANTS whose job it is to show you around.

Now listen,
this is how life
WORKS!

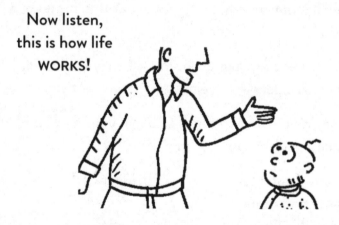

You trust that they know what they're doing because, after all, they've been here LONGER!

You're feeling pretty good about things until the giants start WARNING you about DANGERS.

Watch out for THIS!

Careful of THAT!

Don't go THERE!

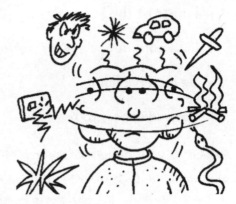

And suddenly this place doesn't feel so FRIENDLY. The more DANGERS they point out to you, the more SCARY this place seems!

And just when you're being your TRUE, NATURAL self, the giants tell you what's WRONG with YOU!

And suddenly you don't feel so good about YOURSELF, either! You thought you could do ANYTHING, but now you're not so sure.

OVERPROTECTION teaches children to:

- Fear life

- Not trust their instincts

- Lose confidence in themselves

- Be hypervigilant

- Rely on others to feel safe

PRAISING your child may seem ENCOURAGING and, by all means, be supportive – but beware of OVERDOING it. EXCESSIVE PRAISE can actually UNDERMINE a child's confidence in the wider world in the long term.

While it is great that you are ENCOURAGING, OVERDOING this can set up some UNREALISTIC expectations that the praise will be UNIVERSAL and ONGOING.

If this isn't the CASE – if the child FAILS or is DISLIKED – the child's self-worth (which relied on receiving praise and being successful), will COLLAPSE.

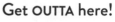

**You think you're
BETTER than us!**

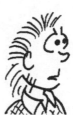

Get OUTTA here!

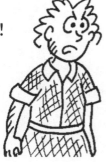

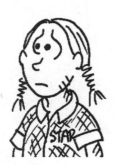

Helping your child embrace and own their
SHORTCOMINGS, as well as their STRENGTHS,
reduces the fear of being 'found out' as LACKING
in some way – a major cause of anxiety.

However, be careful not to SHAME a child through
CRITICISM. Help them to APPRECIATE all the colours
of their personality and INDIVIDUALITY.

**Yeah, I get ANXIOUS.
No BIG DEAL!**

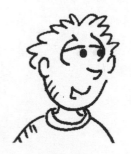

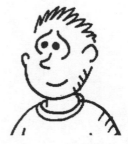

CHAPTER 5

What kids get ANXIOUS about

As mentioned in CHAPTER 1: IS THIS NORMAL?, a certain amount of anxiety is NORMAL in human beings.

BABIES and TODDLERS tend not to worry, which is a BIG clue in itself. We LEARN to be ANXIOUS!

**I'M good. YOU'RE good.
It's ALL good!**

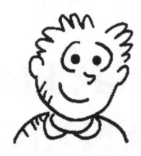

Very young children live very much in the PRESENT. Anxiety is FUTURE-BASED and PREDICTIVE. Worrying requires that we project into the future and IMAGINE possible DANGERS and DISASTERS.

This is why worrying is more common in OLDER CHILDREN, who have a better understanding of themselves and how they fit into the world around them. They also have better language skills to COMMUNICATE what they are worried about.

While EXCESSIVE WORRYING is a key component of anxiety, there are DIFFERENCES in the way that WORRY and ANXIETY are EXPERIENCED.

- WORRY tends to be confined to THOUGHTS, while ANXIETY is usually experienced as a FULL-BODY sensation.

- WORRY tends to be about something SPECIFIC, whereas ANXIETY is more FREE-RANGING and based on ABSTRACT concerns.

- WORRY can lead to PROBLEM-SOLVING, while ANXIETY tends to run in a LOOP.

- WORRY is often more TEMPORARY, while ANXIETY can LINGER.

- WORRY is often based on more REALISTIC concerns, whereas ANXIETY can deviate into IRRATIONAL or EXAGGERATED fears.

Worrying is not necessarily a BAD thing. Worrying over a problem often results in reaching for a SOLUTION and, once reached, the worry eases.

With anxiety, the 'problem' is less clear, and there is a general feeling of UNREST or UNEASE. In this case, the worrying takes on the form of looking for potential 'dangers' to match the fearful sensations, resulting in HYPERVIGILANCE and ongoing AGITATION. This is explored in more detail in CHAPTER 3: WHAT'S GOING ON UPSTAIRS.

While very young children tend not to worry excessively, certain things will trigger FEAR RESPONSES based on SURVIVAL INSTINCTS, such as:

LOUD NOISES

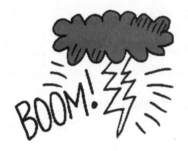

STRANGERS

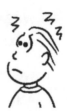
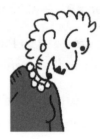

BEING AWAY FROM FAMILY

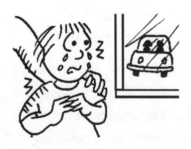

UNFAMILIAR SURROUNDINGS

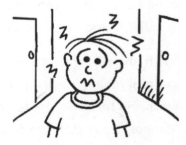

These are NORMAL fears that we still experience as ADULTS to some degree, especially in NEW SITUATIONS.

PRESCHOOLERS start to entertain fearful notions as their IMAGINATION develops. Fears may include:

BEING ALONE

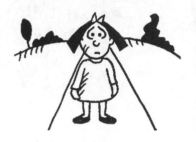

THE DARK

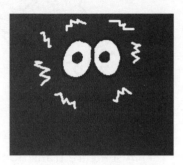

REJECTION

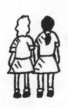 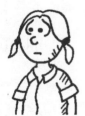

FEAR OF FAILURE

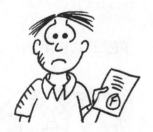

By SCHOOL AGE, fears expand beyond HOME LIFE and into SOCIAL SITUATIONS. Fears include:

PHYSICAL HARM

GHOSTS AND MONSTERS

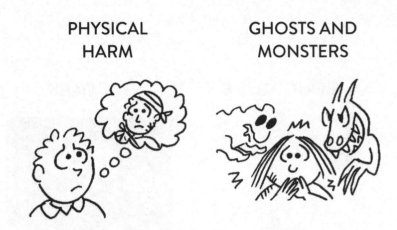

TEENAGERS are transitioning to adulthood and, as such, can develop more complex fears. Most commonly, the issues that are of greatest concern involve OTHERS. Fears for TEENAGERS include:

FEAR OF RIDICULE

NOT FITTING IN

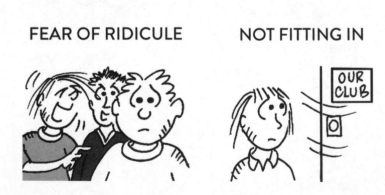

FEAR OF FAILURE

CONCERNS ABOUT THE FUTURE/ WORLD EVENTS

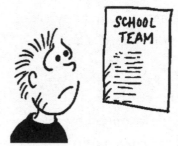

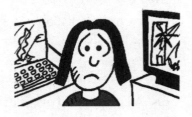

As children get older (and particularly in ADOLESCENCE), fears tend to centre on three main areas:

- FEAR OF FAILURE
- SOCIAL EXCLUSION
- INABILITY TO HANDLE DISCOMFORT

Let's explore these in more detail on the next few pages.

• FEAR OF FAILURE

YOUNG CHILDREN tend not to be particularly
interested in KEEPING SCORE of who WINS or LOSES;
they are more focused on the game itself. They are
quite content to leave a game UNFINISHED and to
resume it later.

They have their own very FLUID concept of SUCCESS
or FAILURE, and this is usually determined by their
immediate personal goals rather than external
standards. Success or failure simply means a DESIRE
is satisfied or not.

A tower of blocks falling down may produce:

TEARS ONE DAY ...

It BWOKE!

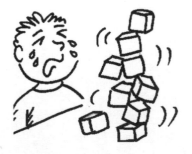

... EXCITEMENT THE NEXT!

YAY! BOOM!

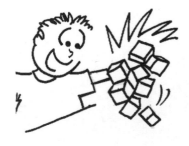

In later years, success or failure tends to revolve around PLEASING ADULTS or fitting into the ADULT WORLD:

GO, Robbie, GO!

You did so WELL, Sweetie!

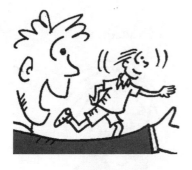
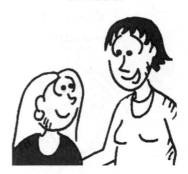

As children enter TEENAGE years, peers may act as SUBSTITUTE AUTHORITY FIGURES whose RESPECT and AFFECTION must be EARNED. If a child is ACCEPTED, this constitutes SUCCESS; if REJECTED, this is interpreted as FAILURE.

• SOCIAL EXCLUSION

Which leads us to the fear of SOCIAL EXCLUSION. When the approval of OTHERS has more currency than approval of SELF, a great deal is invested in others' opinions and attitudes towards us.

In other words, one's own WELLBEING is placed in the care of others, who may or may not have a vested interest in either ESTABLISHING or MAINTAINING that wellbeing.

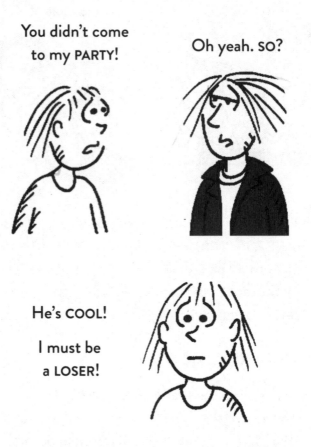

You didn't come to my PARTY!

Oh yeah. SO?

He's COOL!

I must be a LOSER!

If that approval is not forthcoming or is withdrawn, self-worth crumbles. The end result is often not only PAIN but also SELF-DAMNING!

• INABILITY TO HANDLE DISCOMFORT

Here we have the side effects of our modern
24/7 world, where ANYTHING we desire is available
WHENEVER we want it.

Consequently, we have become less and less able to
tolerate DISCOMFORT, such as:

HAVING TO WAIT

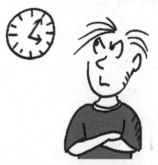

MISSING OUT

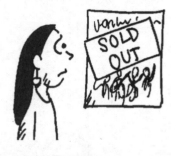

NOT GETTING
IMMEDIATE
ATTENTION

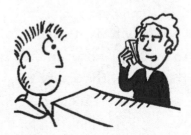

NOT FITTING
THE ACCEPTED
NORM

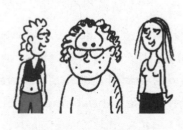

BEING OVERLOOKED

NOT BEING RESPONDED TO IMMEDIATELY
(email, sms, etc.)

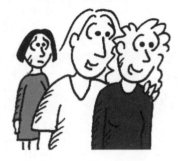

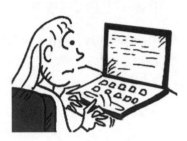

GOING WITHOUT

See my new PHONE?

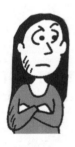

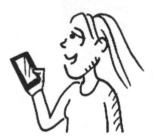

Satisfying a child's every WHIM not only fosters a sense of ENTITLEMENT (which is sure to be disappointed in the wider world) but also deprives the child of the ability to develop essential inner resources such as FLEXIBILITY, PATIENCE and COMMITMENT.

A certain TOUGHENING-UP, which helps us through challenges and crises, can be missing, and this can cause us to OVERREACT to uncomfortable situations – especially uncomfortable EMOTIONS.

The interesting thing about many humans is that rather than becoming more RELAXED and EASYGOING as we get older, we tend to find and create more things to FUSS and WORRY about!

MORTGAGE, DEBT, FAMILY ISSUES, SELF-WORTH ISSUES

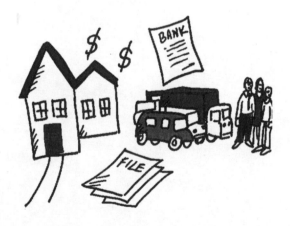

Finding a BALANCE is key to maintaining EQUILIBRIUM. Too much of ANYTHING is still TOO MUCH!

CHAPTER 6

But I DON'T want to!

Handling AVOIDANCE, TANTRUMS and PANICKY moments

Children MANAGE their anxiety in ways that are INSTINCTUAL to them, and AVOIDANCE is usually their first choice.

NO! I WON'T go!

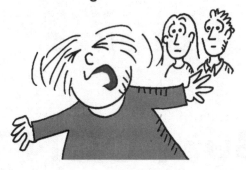

Children will tend to steer away from situations that make them feel anxious, and if facing the situation is UNAVOIDABLE, the child will often resort to CRYING, TANTRUMS, CLINGING or complaining of PHYSICAL SYMPTOMS (such as headaches or tummy aches).

The temptation for the parent is, of course, to GIVE IN.

It's okay, Sweetie, you don't have to go if it's too SCARY!

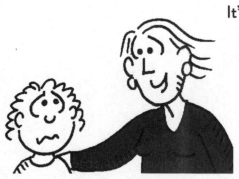

However, while it's difficult to see your child in DISCOMFORT, and you may have the best INTENTIONS, helping your child AVOID these situations only REINFORCES their anxiety.

AVOIDANCE results in the child:

- Assigning ongoing fear to a situation that could be 'NORMALISED' by seeing it through
- Assigning fear to more and more SITUATIONS
- Getting a message that they need ADULT SUPPORT
- Missing out on SOCIALISING and opportunities for RECREATION and LEARNING
- Missing out on developing COPING SKILLS
- Not building necessary RESILIENCE
- Lacking CONFIDENCE in their ability to handle their own fears
- Not learning SELF-REGULATION and SELF-RELIANCE

Well, surely, **FORCING** him is going to make him even **MORE** anxious!

FORCING is not the right approach – ENCOURAGING CHOICE is.

Teaching the child that they have CHOICE and a degree of POWER over the EXPERIENCE and the OUTCOME, even in an unavoidable situation, helps them to feel that they have some CONTROL.

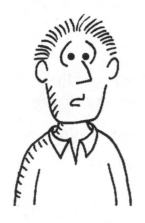

Well, how am I supposed to do that when she's **SCREAMING DOWN THE HOUSE?**

TANTRUMS occur because the child's COMMUNICATION and SOCIAL SKILLS are yet to develop. Their occurrence also means the child is seeking INDEPENDENCE but is still afraid to step away from you.

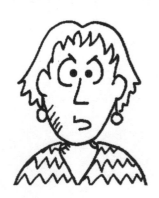

And, if on past occasions a big emotional display has had you running, the child learns that he or she can have INFLUENCE over you.

Unless you want to encourage a NEEDY individual, you need to STEP BACK and let the tantrum roll by until it passes, without becoming emotionally engaged.

So how do I DO that?

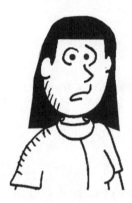

STAY CALM! See the TANTRUM as just a means of expressing FEELINGS. The tantrum in itself is nothing to be worried about, no matter how DRAMATIC it may seem.

It's merely a form of VOCABULARY before the child's language skills fully develop.

Remember, nothing BAD is actually happening!

The child just THINKS it is. Don't CONFIRM that idea.

Here are some STRATEGIES to ward off HYSTERICS:

• HEAD 'EM OFF AT THE PASS

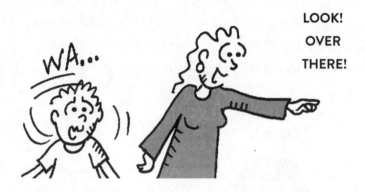

If you see a tantrum on the way, you can DISTRACT your child before it gathers steam.

• TIMING IS EVERYTHING

You're not going to get the best results if you're trying to push your child towards something they are resistant to when they're TIRED or OVERSTIMULATED.

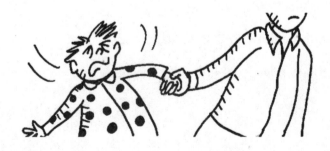

• WAIT OUT THE STORM

Once a tantrum is in full swing, you need to ride it out.
Stay physically close but as emotionally DETACHED
as possible.

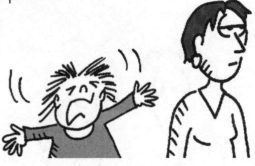

• ACKNOWLEDGE THEIR FEELINGS

This helps your child to reset their feelings and
feel UNDERSTOOD.

Yes, I know it
can feel SCARY.

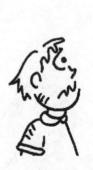
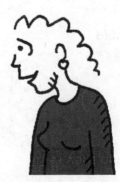

• HELP THEM FIND THE WORDS

Since the tantrum occurs because children don't yet have the WORDS to articulate their feelings, it is helpful to encourage them to NAME their feelings.

Do you feel ...
SCARED?
ANGRY?
SAD?

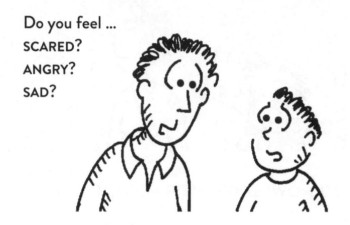

• EXPLORE ALTERNATIVES

Try to IDENTIFY what the child is specifically afraid of and help them to explore OTHER SOLUTIONS.

What ELSE could
you do instead?

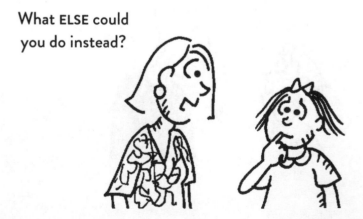

• BE CONSISTENT

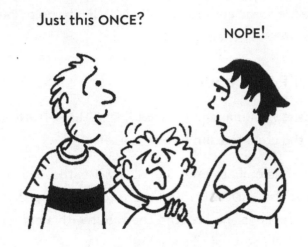

Just this ONCE?

NOPE!

Don't give in SOMETIMES and not at OTHER TIMES –
as this sends a CONFLICTING message.

ADDITIONAL TECHNIQUES

Here are some additional TECHNIQUES to help your child MANAGE their anxiety:

• DEEP BREATHING

To assist with managing anxiety, DEEP BREATHING can help the child to calm him or herself.

Coach the child to take BIG, SLOW breaths, which expand the ABDOMEN. Tell them to gather up their yukky feelings and breathe them out with a big WHOOSH! sound until they feel CALM.

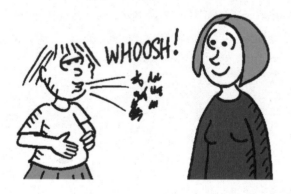

Then have them CLOSE their eyes and clearly VISUALISE themselves SUCCEEDING.

• VISUALISATION

Using IMAGINATION to project forward and VISUALISE a successful outcome in ADVANCE is a great way to soothe fears in the present.

This is most effective when aimed at generating a good FEELING rather than expectations of specific CIRCUMSTANCES determining success.

Say to the child:

> **Now CLOSE YOUR EYES and imagine that you are doing it and it's EASY!**

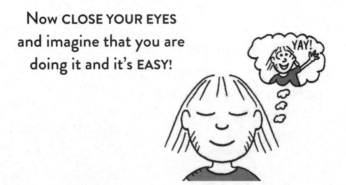

Say to the child:

> **How about you draw me a picture of how BRAVE and CLEVER you will feel?**

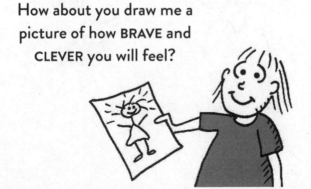

• FEELING THE FEAR AND DOING IT ANYWAY

The idea here is to convey to the child that feeling SCARED isn't proof that there is anything to BE scared of.

Feeling fear about doing something and doing it anyway helps them to realise that while feeling fear may be a component of a new experience, it need not EXCLUDE them from the experience.

I feel SCARED, too, when I try something new! But once I've DONE IT, it's not that SCARY after all!

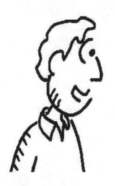 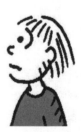

And you can still DO IT even if
you feel scared!

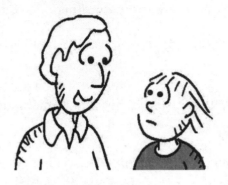

And you'll feel EXTRA GOOD
afterwards, because you still
did it even though you
felt SCARED!

• WORRY TIME

Assigning a specific time to explore your child's
concerns is helpful, and by setting a LIMIT on the
amount of time spent on worries, the worries can then
be seen as SECONDARY, rather than all-consuming.

You may join the child in WORRY TIME to discuss their concerns, or they may prefer to do this alone. Let them decide which they are more comfortable with.

ACTIVITIES that they can do during WORRY TIME may include:

- WRITING DOWN specific worries and thinking up possible SOLUTIONS

- DRAWING their worries, using COLOURS or SHAPES to represent their feelings if the feelings are more abstract

- TELLING their worries to a 'support group' of dolls or stuffed toys

- DOWNLOADING their worries onto objects such as small ROCKS or BEADS, which act as 'worry-cleaners' (often, WORRY BEADS are used in some cultures in a similar way). Once the worries have been 'downloaded', the objects (and therefore the worries) can be disposed of.

Variations of these techniques are also helpful for older children. See CHAPTER 10: TEENAGE ANGST for some additional ways to help teens.

CHAPTER 7

The anxious PARENT

**I suffer from anxiety.
I don't want to PASS IT ON
to my children!**

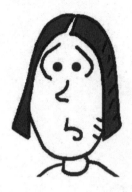

First of all, anxiety is
NOT CONTAGIOUS!

Though there may
be a genetic
PREDISPOSITION in
some cases, most
GENERATIONAL
anxiety is a result of
LEARNED BEHAVIOUR.

In other words, your GENES do not DOOM you to a
certain outcome. You have CHOICE in what you choose
to FOCUS on.

Anxious people WORRY – and WORRY and WORRY!
It goes with the territory, and because of that WORRY,
they are on the ALERT for what could go WRONG –
even if there is no apparent threat.

If you have anxiety and are also a PARENT, your anxiety
can be DOUBLED, because not only do you have your
OWN anxiety to deal with, you have an EXTRA person
(or people) to worry about, too!

And on top of THAT, if you have anxiety, you're going
to worry about PASSING ON your anxiety!

So it is important, for everyone concerned, that you start to get a handle on YOUR anxiety, so that you can show your children how to manage THEIRS.

Notice that I didn't say 'PREVENT' or 'PROTECT YOUR CHILDREN FROM' anxiety. Don't even bother trying to hide it – kids KNOW.

What I did say (and this is important) was 'SHOW YOUR CHILDREN HOW TO MANAGE THEIRS'.

Because, in the end, EVERYONE gets anxious at some time in their lives (and everyone gets DEPRESSED, too) – it's a matter of degree.

And it's not the ANXIETY that's the problem so much as how you HANDLE it.

This simple diagram shows what happens when a problem seems insurmountable:

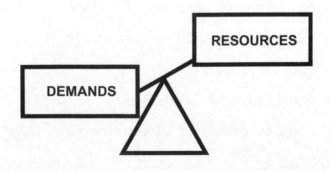

All that's happening here is that the DEMANDS are outweighing the RESOURCES available to deal with the DEMANDS.

In this case, the main RESOURCES for handling anxiety are:

- EDUCATION

- MANAGEMENT SKILLS

- IMPROVED THINKING STYLE

So, let's start with a little EDUCATION about anxiety.

To recap from CHAPTER 2: ANXIETY 101, there are several KEY COMPONENTS to anxiety:

- A tendency to WORRY EXCESSIVELY

- Thoughts are mainly of a NEGATIVE/PESSIMISTIC nature

- Fearful PROJECTIONS into the FUTURE

- EXAGGERATED/CATASTROPHIC fears

- SELF-CRITICISM

- PERFECTIONISTIC tendencies

- Being overly concerned with others' OPINIONS

Another aspect of being an anxious adult is that you could go into CHILD MODE.

What do you mean by CHILD MODE?

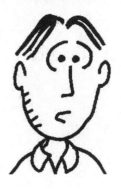

Each of us has an INNER CHILD.

This is the aspect of yourself that, at its BEST, is: PLAYFUL, SPONTANEOUS, OPEN, INQUISITIVE and full of WONDER.

However, when you are ANXIOUS, the less DESIRABLE aspects of the INNER CHILD come to the fore, such as:

- FRETFULNESS

- EXCITABILITY

- EXPECTING THE WORST

- DEPENDENCY

- and a leaning to towards 'MAGICAL THINKING' (believing that one has the power to create DISASTERS or SICKNESS and MOOD CHANGES in others)

Are you suggesting that anxious people are just being CHILDISH?

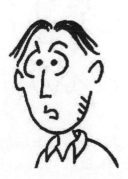

What I am suggesting is that when you are anxious, you feel just as VULNERABLE, POWERLESS and OVERWHELMED as you did as a CHILD, and you tend to REACT to stress as a CHILD might.

Consider the nature of ANXIOUS THINKING, for example:

- *It's too HARD!*
- *I'll NEVER get it right!*
- *What if everyone HATES me?*
- *What if I do something STUPID?*
- *I'm not GOOD ENOUGH!*

Along with SCARING yourself by IMAGINING all that could possibly go WRONG before it's even HAPPENED!

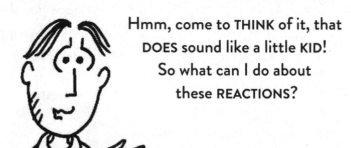

Hmm, come to THINK of it, that DOES sound like a little KID! So what can I do about these REACTIONS?

Just like your own children, your INNER CHILD needs effective PARENTING.

You may not REALISE it, but you ALREADY have an inner 'parent' on board when you CHASTISE, BERATE or BELITTLE yourself.

This is the CRITICAL PARENT, and it is often a voice from the PAST.

You're an
IDIOT!
How could you
be so DUMB?

The role of the CRITICAL PARENT is to prevent you repeating MISTAKES but, in doing so, it tends to convince you that you are NOT GOOD ENOUGH.

Imagine treating your OWN children this HARSHLY! There is no point in being a KIND and CARING parent to your children, if you are being a BULLY to the child inside YOU.

The ANTIDOTE is to become the same SUPPORTIVE, LOVING and NURTURING parent to your INNER CHILD as you are to your own children.

By parenting yourself in a KIND and REASSURING way, you are learning to SELF-SOOTHE in times of distress – a skill that not only serves you but also your children, by example.

Effectively PARENTING yourself means that you become your own:

- CHEER SQUAD
- COMFORTER
- ALLY
- ADVISOR
- CHAMPION

The OUTCOME of this is that you become more INDEPENDENT, RESILIENT and CONFIDENT – skills that you can pass on to your children.

HOW ANXIOUS ARE YOU?

Answer YES or NO to the following questions:

- Do you have trouble sleeping, resting or relaxing?
- Do you see the future as something to worry about?
- Do you see the world as a dangerous place?
- Do you berate yourself for your mistakes?
- Do you need things to be just so before you can relax and enjoy them?
- Do you seldom get enough rest, relaxation and pleasure?
- Do you find changes in physical sensations scary?
- Do you find it difficult to say no to others?
- Do you feel that you give and give but don't get back in return?
- Do you spend more than 50% of your time worrying?
- Can one small upset ruin your whole day?
- If you experience an upset, do you dwell on it for days at a time?
- Do you often re-run old hurts?
- Are you afraid of making a mistake?

- Do you frequently criticise yourself and others?

- Do you worry about what others will think when you make choices or decisions about your own life?

- Do you find it difficult to handle conflict situations?

- Do you live by a lot of rules? (E.g., punctuality, manners, etc.)

- Do you often use (and live by) the terms should, must and have to?

- Do you often feel 'let down' by others or life?

- Do you feel that you are somehow intrinsically bad, wrong or not good enough?

If you answered YES to around 50% or more of these questions, then chances are that you have ANXIETY or, at the very least, you're not very RELAXED about life.

However, it's important for your own and for your children's sake that you do not feel ASHAMED of having anxiety.

Anxiety is particularly common in HIGH ACHIEVERS, so anxiety is often found lurking in the background of some very successful and productive people.

Many of these people have been open about their experience of anxiety, and this has done nothing to damage their careers, so why should you feel BAD about having HIGH SENSITIVITY?

But I don't like my children knowing that I have trouble COPING!

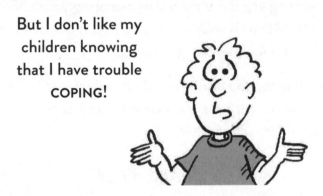

The more you treat your anxiety as a 'dirty little secret', the more you teach your children that anxiety – or, in fact, being VULNERABLE or SENSITIVE – is something to be ASHAMED of. It's NOT.

Do you want your children to be AFRAID of their feelings or RESILIENT to them? You teach by EXAMPLE.

Okay, so how should I handle
my anxiety the BEST WAY
for my children?

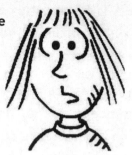

Following are some ways you can bring your children
ON BOARD with your anxiety so that it doesn't seem
ALIEN or FRIGHTENING to them.

In doing so, you also teach them valuable lessons
on how to EMBRACE their own anxiety as being just
another aspect of their PERSONALITY.

SHAME-FREE

Hey kids, I'm feeling
a little ANXIOUS today ...

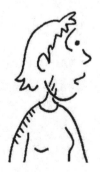
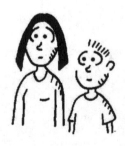

MAKING 'ROOM' FOR ANXIETY

... so I might need
to PACE MYSELF
or take some
TIME OUT ...

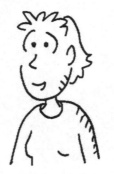

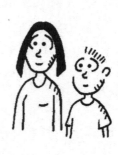

DEMONSTRATING MANAGEMENT

I've been WORRYING
a bit too much
lately, so I'm going
to let that go.

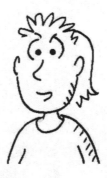

AND RESILIENCE

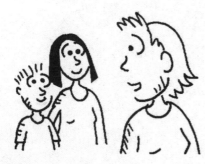

Give me a little while
to SORT THIS OUT
and I'll BOUNCE BACK!

TAKING THE DRAMA OUT OF IT

I've just been hanging out with **IT** a bit too much today!

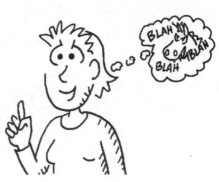

GIVING CHILDREN A HELPFUL ROLE

How about telling me a JOKE?

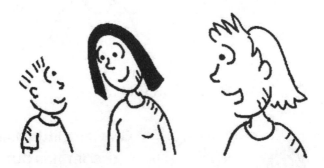

ASKING YOUR KIDS TO BE YOUR 'THOUGHT COACHES'

Hey Dad, you've
COMPLAINED
three times today!

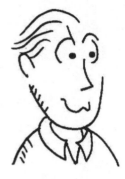
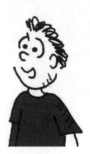

Think of it THIS way: you have the PERFECT OPPORTUNITY to not only learn to effectively MANAGE your own anxiety, but also show your children how to do the SAME!

And, if anxiety is not yet an ISSUE for them, you can be teaching them LIFE SKILLS that help them avoid it becoming an issue!

It has been said that the best gift you can give your children is your OWN happiness, so learning to be more RELAXED, EASYGOING and HAPPY yourself is going to be far healthier for your children than worrying about THEIR emotional welfare.

CHAPTER 8

Getting to KNOW 'IT'

As previously mentioned in CHAPTER 2: ANXIETY 101, each of us has an inner 'NARRATOR', which is that little voice in your head giving a 'COMMENTARY' on just about EVERYTHING!

Most of the time you don't even notice it, as its messages are fairly innocuous and mainly just background mutter.

I'll do the DISHES now ...
or maybe I'll do them later.

Hmm, better watch
those CARBS!

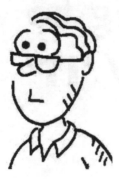
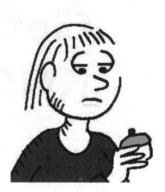

This inner voice is a composite of MEMORIES, BELIEFS, EXPECTATIONS and IMPRESSIONS through which we filter our experience of the world.

This commentary REPORTS ourselves to ourselves!

I'm doing THIS now.

I'm feeling X, Y or Z.

I like THIS,
I don't like THAT.

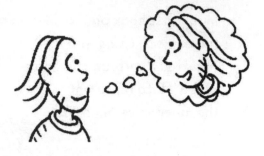

The nature of this 'report' is very dependent on how you FEEL ABOUT YOURSELF.

I'm NOT okay,
so NOTHING'S okay!

I'M okay,
so EVERYTHING'S okay.

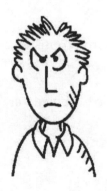

And when you are ANXIOUS, that voice becomes LOUDER, SCARIER, more CRITICAL and delivers only BAD NEWS!

In my first book on
this subject, *Living with IT,*
I created a cartoon character
called '**IT**' to represent
the inner voice of anxiety.

Here he is:

Like many people, at the start of my journey through
anxiety, I thought of **IT** as a kind of MONSTER, who
needed to be DEFEATED. This idea has been reflected
in many children's books on anxiety.

However, depicting **IT** as a fearsome monster can
actually CONTRIBUTE to a child's anxiety.

This is because a 'monster' can be perceived as:

AN OUTSIDER

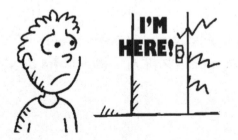

I'M HERE!

IT is one's
OWN creation.
IT is the SELF
at war with SELF.

Anxiety is not caused by EXTERNAL EVENTS but arises
from anxious thoughts ABOUT external events.

PRONE TO SURPRISE ATTACKS

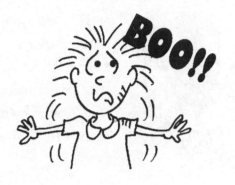

There is always a FEARFUL THOUGHT generating anxiety.

IT does not come from NOWHERE.

To believe that IT attacks RANDOMLY without an associated ANXIOUS THOUGHT creates a sense of being a 'VICTIM' to anxiety, rather than acknowledging the part that your thoughts play in GENERATING IT.

TOO 'BIG' FOR THE CHILD TO HANDLE

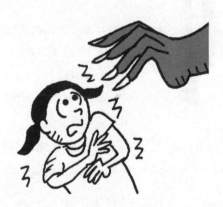

Seeing anxious 'IT moments' as ANNOYING rather than SINISTER brings anxiety down to size and makes it MANAGEABLE.

HAVING MALEVOLENT INTENT

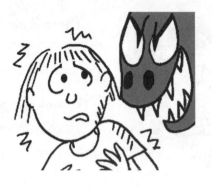

IT is trying to protect SURVIVAL and therefore is acting in one's own BEST INTERESTS.

MUST BE DEFEATED OR ELIMINATED

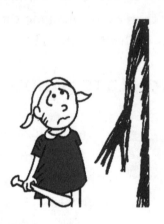

This is an IMPORTANT point – we are not trying to GET RID of **IT** (because **IT** is self!).

Instead, the development of a BETTER RELATIONSHIP with **IT** (self) is needed to restore peace.

The only 'war' taking place is SELF vs SELF, and the only 'ENEMY' to be conquered is one's HARMFUL thoughts.

Over time, as I came to understand **IT**'s true nature, I began to see him in a kinder light.

IT is not a BAD GUY. **IT** is not EVIL. **IT** is not here to PUNISH you for being 'bad' or 'wrong' in some way. And, most importantly, **IT** is not a MONSTER.

Okay, so what is **IT**?

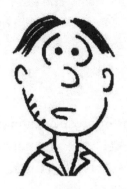

IT is the 'voice' of anxiety – the internal messenger behind ANXIOUS thoughts. He warns of DANGER and acts as an INNER CRITIC to prevent 'DISASTER'.

So how might **IT** fit in with regard to helping my CHILD with his anxiety?

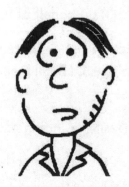

IT is a very helpful device that you can use to help your child both UNDERSTAND and MANAGE their anxiety.

So how do I DO that?

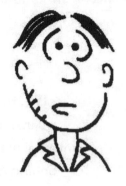

Firstly, it's important that you understand the SUPPORTIVE role that **IT** plays.

As SCARY as the symptoms of anxiety can feel, which can easily but mistakenly be attributed to the torments of some kind of MONSTER, **IT** is actually just an OBEDIENT SERVANT doing his JOB!

IT will do exactly what he is TOLD to do. The only problem is that he tends to do it to an EXTREME.

Remember how we explored the concept of anxiety as being part of our SURVIVAL? **IT** is part of that process – he is looking out for DANGER on behalf of his 'host'.

His sole aim is to keep the host SAFE ... even if to a RIDICULOUS degree! In doing so, **IT** will look for danger even where there is NONE.

IT is simply an UNTRAINED MIND running AMOK!

When **IT** is TRAINED and a COOPERATIVE relationship is established, anxiety is REDUCED.

Tell **IT** that there's something to WORRY about, and he'll go looking for it – and he'll find it!

If there's no OBVIOUS danger, he'll find it in even UNLIKELY places, such as:

BODILY SENSATIONS

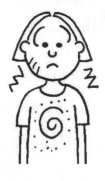

CERTAIN LOCATIONS

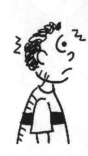 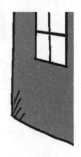

CHANGES IN THE WEATHER

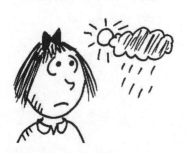

DIFFERENT TIMES OF DAY

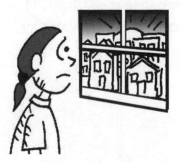

But the KEY AREA that **IT** is likely to find DANGER in is:

OTHER PEOPLE

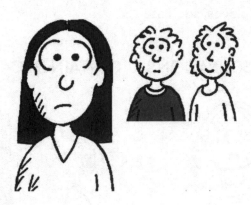

This will present itself as a FEAR OF FAILURE and BEING DISLIKED.

So **IT** tends to be on the lookout for PROBLEMS, and this is governed by THOUGHTS. **IT** is FED by THOUGHTS.

If you think something BAD is happening or MAY happen in the FUTURE, **IT** will seek out all the possible WORST-CASE SCENARIOS to SUPPORT this belief.

What if there's a WAR?

It's everywhere! Look at the NEWS!

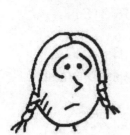
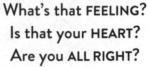

What if I FAINT/ GET SICK/DIE?

What's that FEELING? Is that your HEART? Are you ALL RIGHT?

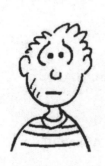
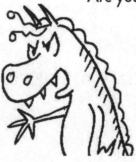

IT doesn't seek PROOF or EVIDENCE, he doesn't REASON, he jumps straight to DISASTER MODE!

IT also indicates that we are in CHILD MODE, as discussed in CHAPTER 7: THE ANXIOUS PARENT.

SIGNS OF BEING IN CHILD MODE

PRONE TO EXAGGERATION

It was HORRIBLE!
I thought I would DIE!

Because you
MISSED THE BUS?

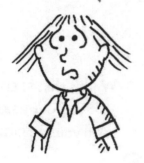
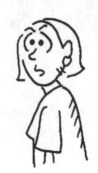

NEEDS OUTSIDE REASSURANCE

I'm okay,
AREN'T I?

I don't know –
ARE you?

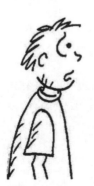
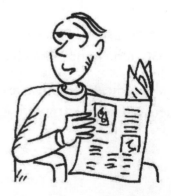

FEAR OF DISAPPROVAL

What if they all
HATE me?

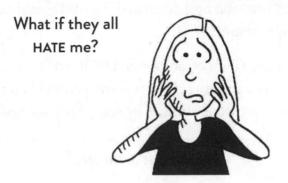

THINKING IN 'ABSOLUTES'

HAVE TO!
GOT TO!
ALWAYS!
NO-ONE!
TOTALLY!
MUST!

'DISASTER' PREDICTIONS

What if someone DIES?
What if I get this
HORRIBLE DISEASE?
What if I MESS
UP EVERYTHING?

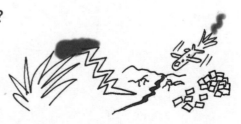

IT also acts as an INNER CRITIC – which is his way of PROTECTING the host from making mistakes that may endanger them.

As a result, **IT** will often demand PERFECTIONISM, a trait common to anxiety sufferers – and you will find that FEAR OF FAILING is a common worry for young people.

I can't get it WRONG!

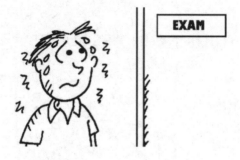

The CRUCIAL point to be understood is that while **IT** can be a hard TASKMASTER, he is only FOLLOWING ORDERS!

And the DETERMINING FACTOR is the THOUGHTS that
IT is being FED.

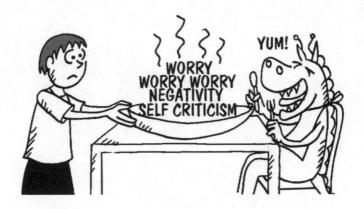

Improve **IT**'s DIET and he will settle down.

Seeing anxiety as an ENTITY, such as **IT**, makes it easier
for children to UNDERSTAND anxiety and develop a
HEALTHIER interaction with the inner monologue that
IT represents.

In the next chapter, we will explore how to do this.

CHAPTER 9

SETTLING
(Little)
IT

I recently started drafting a children's book where I introduced the concept of **IT** as a 'partner' in anxiety, and in particular anxiety management, using a junior version of **IT**.

The most IMPORTANT message about Little **IT** is, as he says:

I AM NOT A MONSTER!

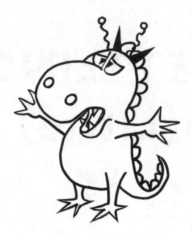

As outlined in the previous chapter, **IT** is simply an OBEDIENT SERVANT, who responds to whatever thoughts he is FED.

If the thoughts are CALM and REASONED, **IT** will be at rest.

But if the thoughts are NEGATIVE and WORRISOME, **IT**'s job is to activate the FEAR RESPONSE that we explored earlier, in order to ensure the safety of the host.

Of course, the SENSATIONS that accompany the FEAR RESPONSE are UNCOMFORTABLE, to say the least, and are therefore often mistaken as a THREAT in themselves.

But they are not. They are merely a PHYSIOLOGICAL reaction to ANXIOUS THOUGHTS.

Feelings are like any bodily sensation – they come and go according to STIMULI. For example, you get goosebumps when there is a sudden shift in TEMPERATURE.

Goosebumps are not a BAD thing; they are just an EFFECT, while the change in temperature is the CAUSE.

The uncomfortable sensations of fear that come with anxiety work in the same way – i.e., CAUSE and EFFECT. The CAUSE is the thought that there is something to FEAR. The effect is the FEAR RESPONSE.

So the first step in settling **IT** is to help your child to experience the BODILY SENSATIONS of fear without adding a particular meaning or FEARFUL STORY to them. DISTRACTION can be helpful in this instance.

It's just your heart going FAST.
Now, have you put away
your SHOES?

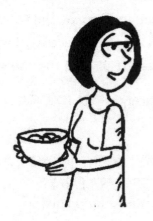 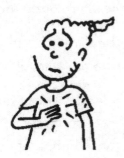

This way, the sensations can pass more quickly, and there are fewer ideas of THREAT associated with them.

Learning to 'sit through' panicky moments, making 'room' for them and allowing them to PASS without DRAMATISING the experience, is an important skill.

However, the greatest focus needs to be on the THOUGHTS that generate the feelings of fear in the first place.

Teaching children to be much more DISCERNING about the thoughts they entertain is key to the MINIMISATION and long-term MANAGEMENT of anxiety.

IT can actually serve as a helpful MONITOR to keep tabs on when thoughts stray into anxious territory.

In other words, if **IT** starts rumbling, this simply means that the thoughts have entered INHOSPITABLE zones.

**Uh oh – IT is waking up!
Now what was I
THINKING about?**

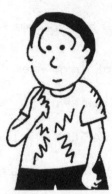

Using **IT** as a device to help children keep their thoughts on track and their anxiety manageable is a great way to also help children become more AUTONOMOUS and EMPOWERED in their self-care.

By working with **IT**, you will be of most help to your child if you:

- Stay CALM and OBJECTIVE

- Downplay the DRAMA

- GUIDE the child to EXAMINE their fears

- Help them to see their fears in PERSPECTIVE

- Allow them to CHOOSE the next step

- Don't push them but GENTLY direct them

- Help them UNDERSTAND that fears are
  NOT FACTS

The AIMS of this work are to help your child to:

- SOOTHE themselves

- Find their own SOLUTIONS

- Gain MASTERY over their thoughts

- Establish and maintain SELF-RESPECT

- Build RESILIENCE

- FEEL the fear and NOT FEAR it

- Distinguish between fearful THOUGHTS and
  physical DISCOMFORT

- Build a HEALTHY RELATIONSHIP with self

- Align with a preferred OUTCOME

We will explore these in relation to **IT** in a moment,
but first INTRODUCE **IT** to your child by explaining that
IT is a part of them who needs HELP to calm down.

When YOU WORRY, **IT** finds things to WORRY about!

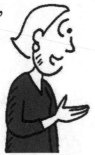

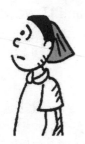

If you think there's DANGER, his JOB is to PROTECT you from it!

Why does he DO that?

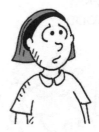

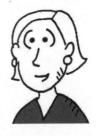

He's just doing what you TELL him to do!

But YOU'RE the BOSS! You get to CHOOSE what you THINK about ...

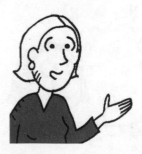

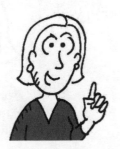

... things that make
you and **IT** WORRY...

BAD
WRONG
SCARY

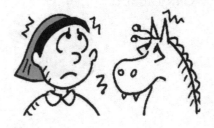

... or things that make
you feel BETTER and
then **IT** can REST!

OKAY
GOOD

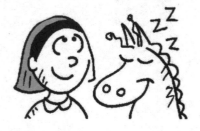

And remember,
Little **IT** is
SCARED, too!

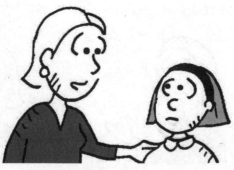

Now introduce the idea of having them DRAW their **IT**.
(I also do this with my ADULT clients, so it's helpful at
any age.)

Shall we MEET **IT**
and see if we can
HELP him?

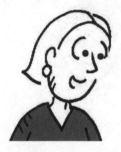 

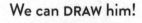

How do we
DO that?

We can DRAW him!

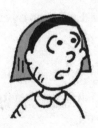 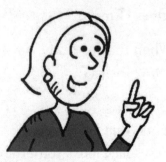

Put out some paper and coloured pencils or crayons.

Have your child CLOSE their eyes and locate **IT** in their BODY. Help the child get a CLEAR PICTURE of **IT** by asking:

Where do you feel IT?

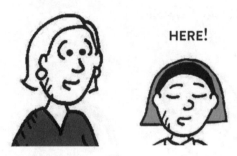

HERE!

'What COLOUR is **IT**'?

'What does **IT** feel like – is **IT** SMOOTH, PRICKLY, HARD, SOFT, SQUIDGY?'

'Does **IT** make a SOUND?'

When they're ready, have them OPEN their eyes and DRAW their **IT**.

Observing hundreds of **IT** drawings over the years, I've found that his appearance is surprisingly consistent. He usually looks something like THIS:

A CONVERSATION between the child and their **IT** is necessary, so they need to have a VISUAL representation of something or someone they can converse with.

If your child draws an **IT** that is not a CHARACTER but a vague SHAPE, ask them to draw whoever is CONTROLLING the shape (even a stick figure will do).

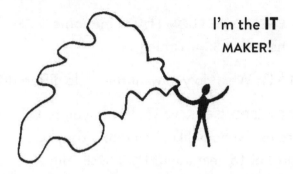

I'm the **IT** MAKER!

Alternatively, for a very young child, you might assign a stuffed toy to represent **IT**, and the child's role is to help to CALM Little **IT** when he's afraid.

Now explain to the child that **IT** is not out to HURT them, but is following COMMANDS, according to what the child THINKS about.

The next step is to open a CONVERSATION between the child and **IT**. The child asks Little **IT** some questions. After each question, have the child CLOSE their eyes and wait for the ANSWER.

Once the answer is received, the child can WRITE it or have you RECORD it, depending on the age of the child.

Here are some examples of a HELPFUL CONVERSATION with **IT**:

CHILD TO IT: How can I get you to calm down?

POSSIBLE RESPONSE FROM IT: Tell me some NICE things, instead of SCARY things!

CHILD TO IT: What do you want me to do differently?

POSSIBLE RESPONSE FROM IT: I need you to be NICER to us! Nobody likes to be told they're BAD or WRONG or to hear about HORRIBLE THINGS that might happen!

CHILD TO IT: But you keep PICKING on me!

POSSIBLE RESPONSE FROM IT: I'm just trying to stop you from making mistakes so that you keep SAFE! You're the one who's scared of getting things WRONG!

CHILD TO IT: Well, I'd like you to tell me in a NICE way. Stop SCARING ME!

POSSIBLE RESPONSE FROM IT: I will, if you stop thinking of things to WORRY about! Then I don't have to watch out for DANGER all the time.

CHILD TO IT: You mean, I decide what YOU do?

POSSIBLE RESPONSE FROM IT: Yes! I just follow your lead! If you CALM DOWN, I can CALM DOWN, because then I know you're all right.

CHILD TO IT: But what if I don't FEEL all right? That's YOU making me feel SCARED, isn't it?

POSSIBLE RESPONSE FROM IT: No – I can't do ANYTHING until you tell me to do it. It's what you're THINKING that makes you feel scared – not ME!

CHILD TO IT: How do I fix that?

POSSIBLE RESPONSE FROM IT: You can tell yourself something that feels BAD, and you'll feel BAD and so will I! But tell yourself something that feels GOOD, and you'll feel BETTER and I won't have anything to do!

Of course, the conversation will vary greatly depending on the age of the child and the depth of their understanding of the role that **IT** plays.

However, allow the conversation to flow spontaneously, then DISCUSS with your child what they have discovered from the conversation.

What about those SELF-CRITICAL thoughts? My child is so HARD on herself!

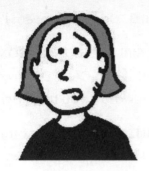

Yes, there are times when **IT** seems to be a BULLY!

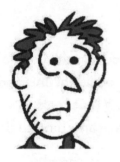

As the Inner Critic, **IT** is seeking to prevent potentially harmful mistakes and avoid attracting EXTERNAL criticism but, typically, he OVERDOES it!

IT is just a bit too STRICT and way too PUSHY!

No-one likes to be told what to do by someone who's BOSSY or who constantly finds FAULT!

Have your child write down the things that **IT** says when he's being CRITICAL. Ask them to think about how HURTFUL these criticisms are.

Now have the child ask **IT** to talk to them NICELY and be ENCOURAGING. Have them write down what **IT** might say if he was being SUPPORTIVE.

But IT says some really SCARY things!

You don't have to BELIEVE him!

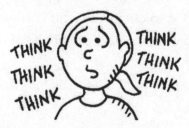

It's not **IT**'s MESSAGES that cause the child to feel scared – it's the INVESTMENT in the ideas of DANGER or WRONGNESS that cause the discomfort.

The child can learn to REFUTE the statements.

But the SCARY THOUGHTS come before I can STOP them!

You can always TUNE THEM OUT!

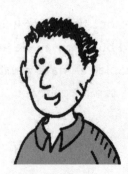

Have the child think of **IT** not as an ENEMY or TORTURER but as an annoying friend who natters on and on, or as a RADIO playing in the background.

The child can also send **IT** 'to his room' where he can natter on all he likes!

The less ATTENTION the child gives to the fearful thoughts, the less he or she FEEDS the fear.

Once the child has begun to form a healthier relationship with **IT** acting as the 'voice' of their anxiety, you can COACH them on how to gain mastery of their THOUGHTS and, in turn, their **IT**.

In simple terms, gaining mastery of thoughts comes down to making a very clear DECISION:

TO FEEL OKAY
(about whatever is going on)

The way we EXPERIENCE something is determined by the way we THINK about it.

It is not the event itself that causes us to feel good or bad but the way we REPORT it to ourselves. This is why people can have greatly CONTRASTING experiences of the same 'reality'.

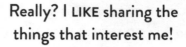

I HATE talking in front of the class!

Really? I LIKE sharing the things that interest me!

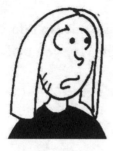

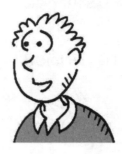

Learning to find POISE and EQUILIBRIUM, even in the most challenging circumstances, is a priceless life skill.

When we learn to RESPOND, rather than REACT, we are also more likely to find a SOLUTION to whatever the problem may be.

PROBLEM

I don't know WHAT to do!

SOLUTION

That's because you can't SEE it from there.

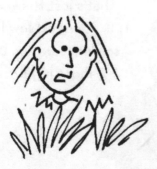

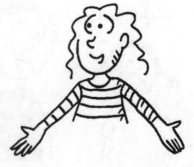

One way to do this is to be less judgmental and rigid in our OPINIONS on matters and to take things (and people) AS THEY ARE.

He's an IDIOT!

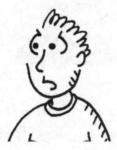

No, he just doesn't do things the way you DO!

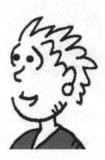

ACCEPTANCE can take the sting out of challenges. It can even ease PHYSICAL PAIN!

Becoming FRUSTRATED, ANNOYED or ANXIOUS about an 'injustice' only ADDS to the distress. We can't always know WHY something has happened in a certain way, but ACCEPTANCE allows us to move on more quickly.

WHY did this happen?

That's just the WAY IT IS, Honey. Now let's see what we can DO about it, eh?

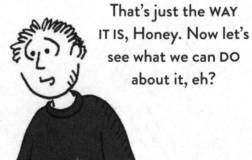

Thoughts PRECEDE and DETERMINE feelings.

When a NEGATIVE or UNSETTLING thought arises, the following questions can be HELPFUL in gaining clarity on the nature of the thought. You can structure the way you present the following concepts to suit the age of the child:

- Is this thought HELPFUL?

  Does thinking this HELP me in ANY way? Does it IMPROVE the situation?

- Is this thought in the HERE AND NOW?

  Is this thought relevant to this present moment, or it is based in the FUTURE or the PAST? If it is not in this present moment, how can it SERVE me in this moment?

- Is this belief a FACT or a GUESS?

  Do I have EVIDENCE to support this IDEA, or is it SPECULATION or even FANTASY?

- Will it make me FEEL OKAY to think this?

  If I continue to think in this way, will I feel more SECURE, CONTENTED or CONFIDENT?

- Will it make me FEEL SCARED to think this? If I want to feel LESS anxious, surely thinking in a way that SCARES me is not going to help me RELAX.

- If I keep thinking this way, am I being NICE to myself?

  Would I say this to a FRIEND or someone I LOVE? If not, then why would I treat MYSELF this way?

- Do I want to feel BETTER or WORSE?

  I get to CHOOSE how I feel. No matter what is happening OUT THERE, I can choose to see it in a way that makes me feel BETTER or WORSE.

- And lastly: will this WAKE **IT** or let him SLEEP?

  If I keep thinking in this way, will I activate the FEAR RESPONSE or help myself stay STABLE?

Here is a simple way of explaining how THOUGHTS affect MOODS.

Imagine that thoughts are BALLOONS. They can either LIFT YOU UP or WEIGH YOU DOWN.

BALLOON FLOATS

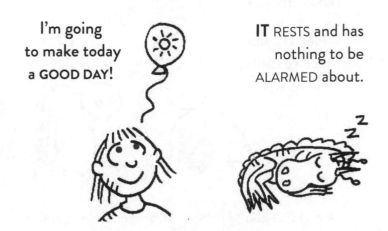

I'm going to make today a **GOOD DAY!**

IT RESTS and has nothing to be ALARMED about.

'LEAD' BALLOON

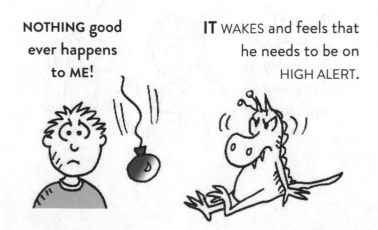

NOTHING good ever happens to **ME!**

IT WAKES and feels that he needs to be on HIGH ALERT.

The **IT** device can be tailored to any age group and modified according to your child's age and personality.

IT can be:

- An annoying, nervous ACQUAINTANCE who simply talks too much and needs to take life less SERIOUSLY.

   Hey IT, you need to CHILL, man!

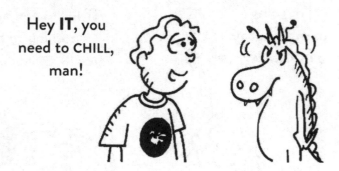

- An OBEDIENT SERVANT who needs clear and HELPFUL DIRECTIVES that come from POSITIVE THOUGHTS.

   Right, IT, I'm going to have FUN today, so I'm going to IGNORE you!

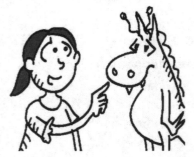

- A PARTNER in anxiety management who acts as a WARNING SYSTEM to alert you when thoughts stray into NEGATIVITY.

WARNING! WARNING!
Yukky thoughts on board!

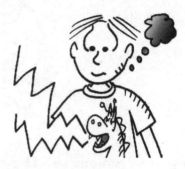

- A GOOD GUY who is LOOKING OUT to protect the child but doesn't know when to STOP.

Thanks, **IT**, but
everything's okay,
    really, it is!

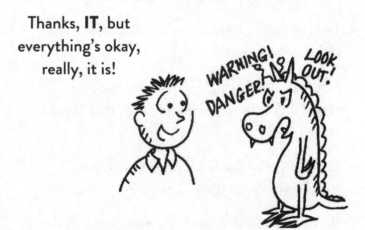

- A frightened INNER CHILD who needs NURTURING, REASSURING but FIRM 'parenting'.

It's okay, Little IT. I'll LOOK AFTER you AND me!

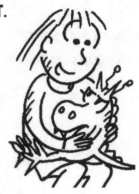

Ongoing conversations with **IT** assist the child to:

- Bring the fear 'DOWN TO SIZE'

- DISTANCE themselves from the anxiety

- Form a more SUPPORTIVE RELATIONSHIP with this aspect of self

- Create a 'PARENTING' dynamic where it is the child's role to soothe **IT** (and, therefore, themselves)

- Build a COOPERATIVE, rather than fearful, relationship with their anxiety

- Be more ATTENTIVE to their thoughts and the resultant feelings

- See the anxiety as a LEARNING TOOL in guiding them back to 'helpful thoughts', therefore building better thinking skills and transforming **IT** from enemy to ally

CALMING TECHNIQUES

Aside from using the **IT** device, here are some more TECHNIQUES that will help your child feel CALMER through anxious episodes. These are especially helpful for very YOUNG children but are applicable to all ages.

• YOGA POSES

The following yoga poses are very helpful in CALMING your child:

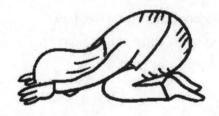

The CHILD POSE is something your child might do INSTINCTIVELY when stressed. This is because it HELPS!

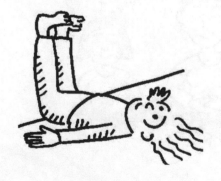

CLIMBING THE WALL is equally calming.

• MEDITATION

Just 15 minutes a day
of meditation can
have a cumulative
effect and is one of
the EASIEST and most
EFFECTIVE tools to
reduce stress.

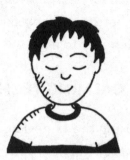

By meditating with your child, you reap the BENEFITS,
too! Simply put on some gentle MUSIC (instrumental
is best), recordings of nature sounds or specially
designed guided meditations (search online for these),
and sit quietly with eyes CLOSED.

Guide your child to simply focus on GENTLE
BREATHING. If THOUGHTS become intrusive, have
them imagine them as being BUBBLES that float to
the surface and eventually pop or drift away.

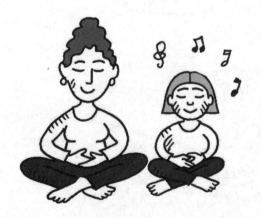

• BABY STEPS

If your child is anxious about trying new things, have them make SMALL, INCREMENTAL steps TOWARDS achieving their goal.

You can list the STEPS involved and have the child mark off those attained.

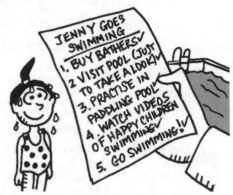

• I'M MUMMY/DADDY

Teaching children to 'PARENT' themselves when anxious can teach them to self-soothe through stressful situations.

Guide them to talk GENTLY and ENCOURAGINGLY to themselves when stressed. This is where a toy representation of **IT** can be most helpful.

What would MUMMY say?

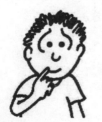

Everything's okay, Darling! You're **ALL RIGHT!** I'm **HERE!**

• SCARY-PROOFING

This is helpful if a child is afraid of GOING TO BED or
of being in a new ENVIRONMENT. Have them take on
the role of 'security officer' and have them arrange
OBJECTS or FURNITURE in such a way as to create a
SAFE PLACE to their own specifications to help them
feel secure.

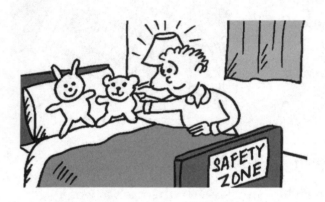

• THOUGHT MASTER

There are many benefits in having the child create a
SUPERHERO version of themselves, such as a 'THOUGHT
MASTER', to manage their anxiety.

Explore with your child the ATTRIBUTES of a superhero
whose role it is to master the use of THOUGHTS in a
way that SUPPORTS the child.

A SUPERHERO has the following attributes:

- Is CALM in a crisis
- Believes in SELF
- Chooses only the BEST for self
- Safeguards own WELLBEING
- Is SELF-RELIANT
- Feels the FEAR and does it ANYWAY
- Is willing to take on new SITUATIONS and CHALLENGES

A THOUGHT MASTER uses GOOD THOUGHTS to fend off DOUBT AND WORRY, build CONFIDENCE, find SOLUTIONS and overcome ADVERSITY.

A THOUGHT MASTER's role is to challenge NEGATIVITY and find the BEST in situations.

Good thoughts are my SWORD and my SHIELD!

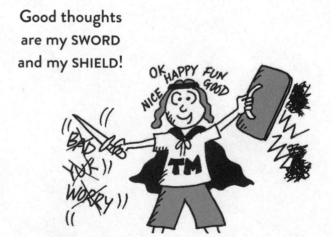

CHAPTER 10

TEENAGE
angst

Naturally, any book addressing children's anxiety needs to include a special section for our beloved but TRICKY teens, doesn't it?

Seemingly overnight, some STRANGE, EXOTIC, INTROSPECTIVE IMPOSTER takes over your child's body and turns them into a STRANGER who looks, sounds and smells familiar but in no way resembles the child who was here yesterday!

And that's just adolescence in GENERAL!

Harder even to contemplate – or accommodate – is the teenager who is ANXIOUS (or depressed).

As stated in the first part of the book, a certain degree of anxiety and depression in teenagers is NORMAL, especially given that they are experiencing such enormous changes, both in their PHYSIOLOGY and MENTAL STATE at this time.

The HORMONES are pumping, and this makes for a very challenging time in anyone's life – both for the child and their parents.

We have covered most bases in the book as to what can be HELPFUL, but this section draws particular attention to major STICKING POINTS when it comes to teenagers.

- **GETTING THEM TO COMMUNICATE** and

- **GETTING THEM TO ACCEPT YOUR HELP**

So let's take a look:

**My teenager is SO anxious,
I can't get THROUGH!**

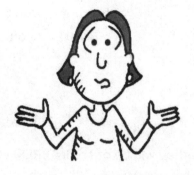

Are there times when
she's NOT anxious?

YES, sometimes.

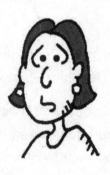

So, essentially, it's not that
the anxiety is an INSURMOUNTABLE
PROBLEM, it's that there's a lack
of CONTROL of the anxiety.

The fact that the anxiety COMES and GOES means that
there is something that governs its coming and going,
and that is THINKING.

As we have explored, it may seem that anxiety
is RANDOM but, in fact, it is determined by the
THOUGHTS that lead to feeling ANXIOUS.

This is the message that you need to UNDERSTAND and CONVEY.

But I try to talk to her and offer suggestions, but she just REFUSES to LISTEN!

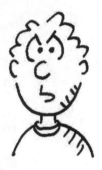

When she's deep IN IT, she simply won't HEAR you.

You can offer remedies, but they will be of NO INTEREST at this point – she would rather JUSTIFY staying stuck.

Think of the times when you feel this way yourself. You find yourself in a DARK PLACE, and the last thing you want to hear is 'helpful suggestions'!

Be POSITIVE!

I'm POSITIVE that you're annoying the HELL outta me!

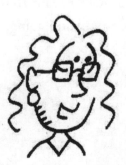

Not only do you NOT HEAR the helpful message, but you also RESENT the messenger!

So what can I DO?

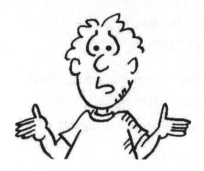

Now and then, you'll be in SYNC – your child will be CALMER and less DEFENSIVE, and THAT is the time to explore some of the OPTIONS that you find in this book.

The BOTTOM LINE is that you can't PUSH anyone (including your child) into GETTING BETTER.

If you try to TAKE OVER this decision for them, it will foster RESISTANCE, and it is less likely that the help will be EFFECTIVE.

No matter how difficult it is to stand by, REACHING OUT needs to come from the one who needs help.

However, you can:

- Let them know you are AVAILABLE to them
- Ask them what they would LIKE to do about the problem
- Leave out helpful materials such as INFORMATION leaflets

- ACKNOWLEDGE their feelings
- COACH them through difficulties
- ENCOURAGE them to find their own solutions

If and when they are WILLING to reach out, here are a few approaches that can be HELPFUL.

Also, remember to revisit the techniques discussed in CHAPTER 6: BUT I DON'T WANT TO! and CHAPTER 9: SETTLING (LITTLE) **IT** to help your child manage their anxiety:

- DEEP BREATHING
- VISUALISATION
- FEELING THE FEAR and DOING IT anyway
- YOGA
- MEDITATION
- and several more!

• HAVE THEM WRITE DOWN THE FACTS

My name is Joel. I have a test tomorrow.

I'm scared that I'll fail.

I think that if I fail ... (add extreme thoughts here).

If I fail it will mean ...

• THEN HAVE THEM REFUTE THEIR FEARS

I've studied for it.

I can only do my best.

I will either pass or fail.

If I fail, I'll deal with it.

I've passed before.

*Failing a test does not mean anything
except that I've failed one test.*

If I fail, I will still be me.

• HAVE THEM WRITE IT AS THEY WANT IT TO BE

*(This needs to be written in present tense and stated
as a 'fact'.)*

My name is Lily.

I am really good at this subject.

I pass tests easily.

I am calm when I do this test.

I pass this test.

Then have them close their eyes and clearly VISUALISE themselves SUCCEEDING. See page 93 for more information about this technique.

VISUALISATION works best when the desired FEELING is called to mind, rather than trying to visualise specific circumstances.

- **BETTER NEXT TIME**

  How can you make it come out DIFFERENTLY next time?

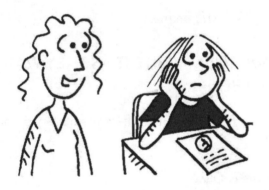

- **GRATITUDE JOURNAL**

Anxiety can cause your child to see only what is LACKING. By fostering GRATITUDE through a daily focus, they learn to IDENTIFY and APPRECIATE that, for all the things that may seem WRONG, there are numerous things in life that provide us all with COMFORT, NOURISHMENT and SUPPORT.

In the GRATITUDE JOURNAL, have your child:

- List 3 things that are WRONG

- Then list 5 things that are RIGHT

With regard to WORLD AFFAIRS, it is interesting to note that the child's main fears centre on issues around IDENTITY and WORTH, and feeling ILL-EQUIPPED to handle whatever 'bad' thing might be coming.

My son is very anxious about the STATE OF THE WORLD! He's very worried about the FUTURE!

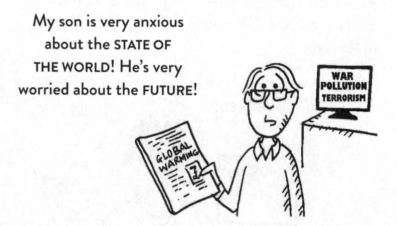

In other words, these fears are about a lack of CONFIDENCE, rather than EXTERNAL FACTORS.

While concern about world events such as WAR, CLIMATE CHANGE, CURRENT CRISIS and OVERPOPULATION are REASONABLE fears, anxiety, by and large, is based on UNREASONABLE fears, or reasonable fears being EXAGGERATED to the point of being unreasonable.

This UNREASONABLE (i.e., without REASON) anxiety focuses on 'What if?' speculations and can manifest as generalised, free-floating ANGST.

If your child is afraid of world events, have a candid talk to them. Don't SUGAR COAT it, but put it in PERSPECTIVE.

Here are some thoughts to consider.

The world has always been MESSY –and it will never be PERFECT. Humans will ALWAYS have CONTRAST. It's how we EXPAND.

Everything's SORTED ...
now I'm BORED!

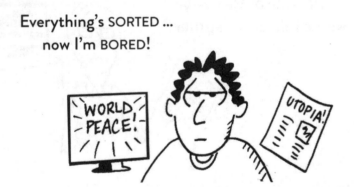

Without CHALLENGES and CONTRASTS, there would be no ADVANCEMENTS, NEW SOLUTIONS or BREAKTHROUGHS.

It's easy to invest in and foster an idea that the world has gone to the dogs, but that's because we're more EXPOSED to world events than ever before, and the media tends to focus on SENSATIONALISM. BAD NEWS is always more INTERESTING!

But for every BAD NEWS story, there is a story of GENEROSITY, KINDNESS and SELFLESSNESS.

In fact, many INJUSTICES and INHUMAN ACTS that have been swept under the carpet for decades have now been brought to light and have led to NECESSARY CHANGES.

- **SELF-WORTH**

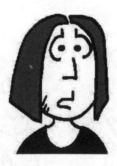

SOCIAL MEDIA has caused my daughter to be completely hung up about her APPEARANCE.

Here is a SELF-WORTH exercise.

1. Think of someone who loves you NO MATTER WHAT.

2. Imagine that you can STEP INSIDE them and that you're looking through THEIR EYES at YOU.

3. WRITE down all the things IN YOU that they see.

4. Now step back into yourself and CLAIM these things for YOURSELF.

My boy is an
EXCELLENT student,
but he is constantly
afraid of **FAILING**!

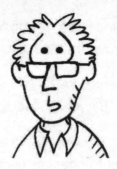

Help to curtail PERFECTIONISM in your child. Explore
FAILURE as being a HEALTHY part of life.

What if you always
had a **PERFECT SCORE**?
Wouldn't that get
BORING?

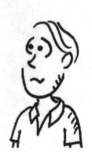

• DEALING WITH BULLIES

What about **BULLYING**?
There is some **TERRIBLE**
ABUSE online!

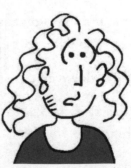

There are 3 basic rules for dealing with BULLIES, whether in PERSON or as internet TROLLS:

1. DON'T REACT.

2. STAND UP for yourself.

3. TELL someone/report it.

There is a lot of helpful online material on DEALING with bullying that you could explore, or speak to your child's school to get their ADVICE.

Consider exploring the following concepts with your child:

WE TEACH OTHERS HOW TO TREAT US

**What MESSAGE do you think
you might be sending that
makes them BULLY you?
How can you CHANGE that?**

DON'T BUY INTO IT

Bullies may APPEAR to be in POWER, but the OPPOSITE is true. No-one who is truly empowered needs to BULLY.

If the child has healthy SELF-ESTEEM, bad behaviour in others is not seen as a reflection of themselves, and they can shrug it off.

A child can do a lot to PREVENT bullying by having a greater sense of their own WORTH.

CRITICISM is only HURTFUL if it feels TRUE in some way.

• VISIBLE EXPRESSIONS OF ANXIETY

Here are some common ways that anxious children (and adults) show signs of having anxiety:

**My child is SO FUSSY!
She checks and rechecks
EVERYTHING! Is this anxiety?**

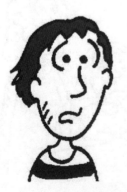

This might be OCD (Obsessive Compulsive Disorder), which is an anxiety-related disorder.

Other anxiety-related behaviours can include:

PICKING AT SKIN

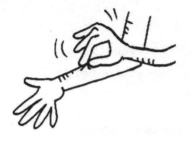

PULLING OUT HAIR

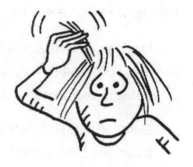

NAIL-BITING

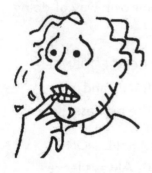

SOCIAL AVOIDANCE

As UNPLEASANT and even DISTRESSING as the
above may be to witness, they are nonetheless
SELF-SOOTHING behaviours in response to anxiety.

If anxiety is reduced, there is no need for the
behaviours. If the behaviour is EXCESSIVE, your child

may require PROFESSIONAL HELP to address their anxiety.

Above all, you can be of most help to your teen by making room for them to:

- FIND THEIR OWN SOLUTIONS – even if that means IGNORING some things you're not entirely comfortable with.

- BUILD RESILIENCE – this can only happen by bouncing back from CHALLENGES and may involve tolerating some discomfort.

- EXPLORE THEIR INDIVIDUALITY – they are their OWN PERSON and have their own way of doing things.

- LEARN THAT CHOICES HAVE CONSEQUENCES – this involves TRIAL AND ERROR, and UNAVOIDABLE MISTAKES in the process.

- EXPRESS THEIR FEELINGS IN A SAFE, NON-JUDGMENTAL ENVIRONMENT. Always leave the door open for them to CONFIDE in you. Let them know that you are ready to LISTEN whenever they are ready to talk.

And, no matter how tricky this time may be, LOVE them through it. They'll come out the other side one day!

A FINAL WORD

As I mentioned at the start of the book, it's important to SEEK HELP from a qualified PROFESSIONAL if your child needs individualised SUPPORT to assist with overwhelming anxiety. A therapist can help your child work through ongoing issues and help manage their anxiety.

Hopefully, you are now armed with a kitbag of UNDERSTANDING and TECHNIQUES not only to help your little worrier back on their feet, but also to arm them with a sword and shield of POSITIVITY that will see them fend off those worries and send them packing!

If so, my work here is done.

Over to you now, with my best wishes.

Also by
Bev Aisbett ...

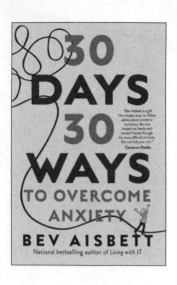

30 DAYS 30 WAYS
TO OVERCOME ANXIETY

From Bev Aisbett, Australia's bestselling anxiety
expert and author of the classic national bestseller
Living with IT, comes a proven and practical workbook
to help people manage their anxiety, with simple
daily strategies for work and for home.

Based on the exercises Bev has been teaching
and writing about for the past twenty years,
30 Days 30 Ways to Overcome Anxiety provides
clear, simple daily building blocks to help people
manage their anxiety and assist in recovery.

Designed to be carried in handbags or backpacks
as a daily companion, this is a highly approachable,
concise, practical and, above all, proven method
of overcoming anxiety.

ISBN: 978 1 4607 5465 8

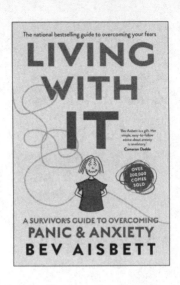

LIVING WITH IT:
A Survivor's Guide to Overcoming Panic & Anxiety

Panic attacks — approximately 5% of the population will experience them at sometime or another. Seemingly coming from nowhere, the dread of having an attack itself transforms the ordinary world of everyday life into a nightmare of anxiety and suffering.

In this refreshing and accessible guide, Bev Aisbett, a survivor herself of Panic Syndrome, tells us how panic disorders develop and how to recognise the symptoms. With the aid of her inimitable cartoons, she covers topics such as changing negative thought patterns, seeking professional help and, ultimately, learning skills for recovery. *Living With IT* provides much needed reassurance and support, leading the way out of the maze of panic with humour and the insight of first-hand experience.

ISBN: 978 1 4607 5717 8

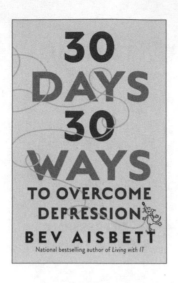

30 DAYS 30 WAYS
TO OVERCOME DEPRESSION

When you're suffering from depression, sometimes it's as much as you can do to get out of bed, let alone read a book. But this just isn't any other book. This is a practical day-by-day workbook, with clear, simple daily building blocks and exercises designed to help pull you out of the inertia of depression. It's a highly approachable, concise and, above all, practical way to help manage depression.

Featuring all-new material from experienced counsellor and bestselling author of the self-help classics *Living with IT* and *Taming the Black Dog*, Bev Aisbett has based this book on many of the exercises she has been teaching and writing about for the past twenty years to help people manage their depression.

ISBN: 978 1 4607 5810 6

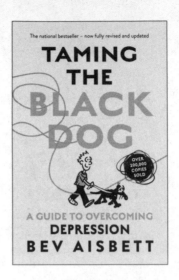

TAMING THE BLACK DOG:
A Guide to Overcoming Depression

Don't want to get out of bed in the morning?

Feeling as though the light is fading at
the end of the tunnel?

You may be suffering from depression, a condition
Winston Churchill referred to as the 'Black Dog'.

Now expanded and fully updated, *Taming the Black
Dog* is a simple guide to managing depression, which
an estimated 1 in 5 people will suffer in one form or
another at some time in their lives. Modelled on
Bev Aisbett's successful *Living with IT*, *Taming the
Black Dog* has a unique blend of wit and information,
and is an invaluable guide for both chronic sufferers
of depression as well as anyone with a
fit of 'the blues'.

ISBN: 978 1 4607 5696 6